NCLEX-RN Practice Questions to become a Nurse!

Voted Top Nursing NCLEX-RN Prep Book with Over 400 Questions and Detailed Answers with Explanations

Alex Ryan & Marie Kaye

Table of Contents

I. NCLEX Exam One

QUESTIONS:

1. A 32 years old, female, on hospitalization in a 5-patients ward, on oxygen therapy, with no signs of any distress during the nurse's rounds. Suddenly, alarms came from the area, the other patient noticed that this female patient monitor is beeping. Upon checking, the nurse saw a 87% oxygen saturation, what should be the first action of the nurse?

   a. Administer 100% oxygen and suction the patient.

   b. Let the patient sit up straight and let her do deep breathing.

   c. Elevate the head part of the patient, ask her to do DBE and coughing exercises.

   d. Increase oxygen administration, continually do routine assessment and suction for secretions.

2. A nurse knows that a patient having a 95-100% SPO2 does not generally requires invasive intervention. However, some conditions may exhibit a normal range of SPO2 even experiencing a fatal condition. The following may result to an abnormal SPO2, except:

a. Anemia

b. Reynauld's Disease

c. Hypovolemia

d. Diabetes

3. A patient on ventilator attached to his ET tube became restless and has shown ineffective ventilation. It is also noted the patient was difficult to ventilate. The first response of the nurse is to call the RT. Upon inspection there is no physical or any mechanical causes found, which means the ventilator is working properly. The ET tube is checked for placement and found to be properly attached. What should be the next action?

a. Recommend sedating the patient.

b. Ask the doctor to change the ventilator machine of the patient.

c. Reposition the patient to check for obstruction.

d. Disconnect ET tube from the ventilator and connect it to BVM and manually ventilate the patient.

4. The staff nurse is supervising a newly hired nurse in caring for a patient on a ventilator. The new nurse heard an alarm on the ventilator and went to check it right away. The ventilator indicated a low-pressure alarm. The staff nurse knows that the new nurse is performing the right assessment on the ventilator when she checks the:

a. Secretions of the patient and suctions the secretions.

b. Ventilator tubes for any disconnections or leaks.

c. The patient, if he is biting the tube.

d. ET tube for placement, as well as the cuff for reinflation.

5. A 60 year old patient with a 2-day old tracheotomy tube became restless and assessment shows that the tracheotomy has been dislodged. The nurse immediately notified the physician and the RT. What should the nurse perform next?

   a. Ask the LPN to hold the tracheostomy tube in place while you get the suction and other equipments needed.

   b. Prepare the BVM immediately.

   c. Open the tracheostomy tube with a sterile hemostat, suction catheter or sterile gloved finger.

   d. None, because only a trained personnel should replace the tracheotomy tube.

6. Upon nursing rounds, the incoming nurse sees continuous bubbling in the water seal chamber of the patient's chest tube. According to what the nurse's knowledge, this is indicative of:

   a. This is practically normal as it is collected to the patient's lungs.

   b. This means that the lungs are already filled with air, no more secretions.

   c. This signifies that there is an air leak in the system.

   d. This indicates that the chest tube should be replaced.

7. The patient with chest tube reported that his side is always wet. The nurse checks that the water seal chamber has no air leaks and no presence of secretions. Inspecting the insertion site reveals that the tube is almost hanging at his side, and would fall if the dressing is not present. What would should the nurse do?

   a. Notify the RT or physician STAT.

   b. Stay with the patient and monitor for signs of respiratory distress.

   c. Tape three sides the wound dressing, leaving one open for air to escape.

   d. Cover the chest tube insertion site with a sterile occlusive dressing.

8. A nurse from the pediatric unit was transferred to the medical unit as a floater. The head nurse at that time assigned her to feed all the patients in the left wing of the ward. All the patient has a nasogastric tube in place. She is correct in saying that nasogastric tubes are these, EXCEPT for:

   a. Checked for placement before every feeding.

   b. Used to feed the patient and the markings indicate the placement.

   c. Used for suction and irrigation and are called Levine tubes.

   d. On feeding the patient Salem sumps, air vent should be kept open.

9. The 42-year old male patient, on NGT complains of having chest pains 30 minutes after the nurse feed him. Checking his records, the nurse found out that he has a history of CHD. What is the main cause and nursing intervention that should be done?

   a. Check for the pulse rate and blood pressure, the pain must be caused by his disease.

   b. Place the patient in a semi-fowler's position, and verify the placement of the tube.

   c. Administer nitroglycerin as an emergency drug.

   d. Withhold the feedings, review his medications and notify the physician.

10. An IV Therapy Nurse needs to take a blood sample from a 17 year old female for routine analysis. The patient has an IV treatment on her left hand. She requested that she wants the blood taken from her left arm as she is using her right in all her activities. Which response of the nurse is correct in dealing with the patient:

   a. "I should collect from your right hand because the blood in your left hand is mixed with IV fluid."

   b. "I cannot collect from your left hand because blood samples should be taken from the dominant hand."

   c. "Okay, I will get the sample in your left hand, but it should be on an area higher from the IV site."

   d. "I will need to ask you to sign in the nurses' notes that you prefer the left arm."

11. The nurse observing an RT in collecting a blood sample for Blood gas test noticed that the RT asked the patient to clench and release is fist while he press the radial part of the patient. This test is known as:

    a. Radial Blanch Test

    b. Allen Test

    c. Arterial Puncture Test

    d. Arterial Pressure Test

12. The nurse knows that the family member of the patient understood the importance of 24 hour urine collection when:

    a. He keeps all the urine for the entire duration, especially the first void.

    b. He places all the collected urine in a container filled with ice or in a refrigerator.

    c. He freezes all the collected urine and record the date and time each time the bottle is filled.

    d. He should allow the patient to drink lots of fluid and submit only the selected bottles.

13. There is a need for a sputum sample on a 36-year old patient, the nurse gave the correct instruction when the patient says the following, EXCEPT:

    a. "I need to take 2-3 deep breaths before I cough."

    b. "I need to perform oral hygiene prior to specimen collection."

    c. "I need to collect sputum 1 day after drinking my antibiotics."

    d. "I should directly spit in the container."

14. The nurse doing her rounds noticed a patient with an abnormal breathing pattern. She noted that at times the patient is breathing deep, at times breathing shallow, there are also moments of cessation of breathing. The nurse that this kind of breathing is caused by a neurological problem, also known as:

    a. Apneustic

    b. Kussmaul's

    c. Hyperventilation

d. Cheyenne-Stokes

15. A nurse is doing a physical assessment of the abdomen of a patient. With her knowledge, the correct order of assessing the abdomen is:

a. Percussion, Palpation, Inspection and Auscultation.

b. Inspection, Palpation, Auscultation and Percussion.

c. Inspection, Auscultation, Percussion and Palpation.

d. Auscultation, Inspection, Percussion and Palpation.

16. A saleslady complained of pain in her leg when she tries to flex it. The pain continued from work until she reached home. She can no longer endure the pain and seeks medical consultation. The nurse in the ER Department assesses her legs and noticed venous distention, and cold skin. This reinforced her assessment that the patient is suffering from what condition:

a. Edema of legs

b. Venous stenosis

c. Reynauld's Disease

d. DVT

17. The wife of a diabetic patient approached you because she is concerned about the edema in her husband's feet. She wonders if it will heal. As the nurse, you explained the reason of having edema and the interventions to be done. She also reported that she saw cracks in the area. This is indicative of:

a. Healing of the edema

b. Early signs of gangrene

c. Dryness of the skin

d. Scratching of the patient in the area.

18. In caring for a bedridden patient in home care, the nurse knows the importance of positioning and logrolling the patient. She instructs the relatives of the patient in order to acquire their cooperation. After a month of home care, the relatives brought the patient back to the hospital because they saw an eschar on the coccyx area and was alarmed about it. The nurse knows that this is:

   a. Stage I of pressure ulcer.

   b. Stage III pressure ulcer.

   c. Stage V of pressure ulcer.

   d. Stage II of pressure ulcer.

19. During a physical examination, the nurse is testing for a man's coordination. She asks him to stand with feet together, eyes closed for 10 seconds. For a positive result the patient should become unstable. This test is called:

   a. Romberg's test

   b. Rapid alternating movement test

   c. Proprioception test

   d. Point-to-point movement test

20. A patient with a GCS score of 15 indicates that the patient is very good, with no signs of brain injury. A score of 3-8 indicates severe brain injury. What does a score of 10 indicate?

   a. Mild brain injury

   b. Moderate brain injury

   c. Comatose

   d. Inappropriate behavior

21. A 16 year male was brought to the hospital due to hyperthermia that started two days ago. The nurse attending to his case will start her planning. Which of the following is the correct plan of care?

   a. Environment manipulation by increasing air circulation in the room.

b. Restriction of fluids to 2,000 ml in a day.

c. Continuous monitoring of body temperature every two hours.

d. Encourage activities of daily living to help the patient cope with the disease.

22. A 27 year old kitchen crew was cleaning the table top when his right sleeve caught fire and burned his right arm. The nurse in the ER Department is cleaning the wound and she noticed the facial grimaces of the patient. Which of the following nursing intervention should be included for reducing pain?

a. Elevate the patient's arm to decrease the venous return to the heart.

b. Apply warm packs to reduce edema.

c. Keep the wound wet and clean.

d. Administer anti-inflammatory agents as prescribed.

23. Anna, a 37–year old office clerk, went to the Outpatient department with complaints of urinary dribbling. The nurse knows that this altered urinary pattern can be corrected with the help of:

a. Asking the patient to maintain the newly inserted indwelling Foley catheter for one day bladder training.

b. Instruct how to perform Kegel's exercise and ask her to perform it at home.

c. Instruct the patient on the Valsalva maneuver to aid her urinary problem.

d. Encourage the use of pads or diaper for the patient.

24. Mr. Bart, a 45-year old business owner, is now being discharged from the acute care setting. Which of the following should be included in the nurse's discharge plan of care?

a. Instruct in ways to reduce stress.

b. Evaluation of home environment and coping techniques.

c. Maintaining personal cleanliness such as skin care measures.

d. Encourage participation in activities of daily living.

25. Mar, a student nurse is given the assignment of taking care of patient Leo, 39 years old father of 2 children. During an interview and assessment, Mar noticed that Leo exhibits facial grimaces. Mar asked him to rate his pain on the pain scale of 1 (no pain) and 10 (worst pain). Leo rated 8/10. Which of the following interventions shows that Mar understands the meaning of the pain scale?

    a. Ask if the patient has pain medication and tell him to drink it.

    b. Instruct the patient to follow on how to do guided imagery.

    c. Use therapeutic conversation techniques to alleviate pain.

    d. Assess the reason of the pain before administering medication.

26. The blood Chem of a patient revealed potassium of 1.7mEq. During the interview, the patient said that she suffered from vomiting and diarrhea prior to hospitalization. Which of the following food should the nurse include in the plan of care?

    a. Whole wheat bread and apple

    b. Milk products, liver and green leafy vegetables

    c. Nuts and meat products

    d. Orange juice and banana

27. At the end of his shift, Nurse Mike is totalling the intake of his patient on a clear liquid diet. He noted that the patient had 8 Oz. of fruit juice, 950 ml of water, 1 cup of broth, and 800ml of normal saline solution. Her output is 1,600 ml of urine during the shift. How many ml is the patient's total intake?

    a. 2,740

    b. 2,430

    c. 2,470

    d. 2,340

28. Joe, the nurse on duty is taking the blood pressure of the patient when he noticed carpopedal spasm after the cuff was inflated. Lab results also revealed a serum calcium of 2.3 mEq/L. These results indicate that the patient is:

   a. Hypercalcemia with positive Chvostek's sign

   b. Hypocalcemia with positive Chvostek's sign

   c. Hypercalcemia with positive Trousseau's sign

   d. Hypocalcemia with positive Trousseau's sign

29. A 56-year old male patient with a history of chronic obstructive pulmonary disease has the following ABG result: PO2 – 60 mmHg, pCO2 – 55 mmHg. To improve the patient's ventilation, which of the ABG values are the primary stimulus for the patient's breathing?

   a. High pCO2

   b. Low pCO2

   c. High PO2

   d. Low PO2

30. A 17 year old student had a blood result of 0.8 mEq/L of magnesium. The nurse knows that the patient is at risk and includes which of the following interventions?

   a. The patient is at risk of infection and teaches the importance of preventing infection.

   b. The patient is at risk injury and initiates seizure precaution.

   c. The patient is at risk of blood problems and will avoid using a tourniquet in drawing blood.

   d. The patient is at risk of cramps and should encourage early ambulation.

31. Alex has a serum electrolyte test with the following results: Na – 138mEq/L, K – 6.5mEq/L, Chloride 102mEq/L. What would the nurse anticipate as the medication the physician will prescribe?

   a. Potassium supplements

   b. Sodium supplements

c. Kayexalate

d. Calcium gluconate

32. A patient in the medical ward is prescribed by the doctor to take furosemide BID P.O. and digoxin O.D. The nurse knows that he should monitor which serum electrolyte?

    a. Calcium level

    b. Sodium level

    c. Potassium level

    d. Magnesium level

33. Mrs. Agnes, 33-year old pregnant, went to her first trimester check-up. During the interview, she told the nurse that this is her third pregnancy. Her second pregnancy did not complete, and her oldest is 5 years old. The nurse knows that Mrs. Agnes has a gravida of:

    a. 1

    b. 2

    c. 3

    d. 0

34. Looking at the records for Mrs. Agnes on question 33. Her GTPAL is:

    a. 31013

    b. 31011

    c. 32012

    d. 31012

35. Mrs. Agnes completed the full term and gave birth to a baby boy. The attending doctor told her that her baby is LGA. Unable to ask the doctor, Mrs. Agnes asked the nurse. The nurse knows that LGA stands for:

    a. Low for Gestational Age

    b. Less than the Gestational Age

c. Large for Gestational Age

d. Left for Gestational Age

36. Liza, pregnant of her first child went to the family planning clinic, and Marie is the nurse in charge. Liza is so excited about her pregnancy and asks Marie a lot of questions. One of the questions is the development of her baby's organs. Marie knows that organogenesis starts:

a. Upon conception

b. On the first week

c. On the second week

d. On the third week

37. In predicting Liza's due date of pregnancy, the nurse asks for her first day LMP. Liza replied May 20, 2015 The nurse knows that using Nagele's Rule it will be:

a. March 27, 2016

b. February 27, 2016

c. March 7, 2016

d. February 7, 2016

38. A couple went to the family planning clinic for a check-up. The husband wants to know the different developments that happen in her wife's womb. As the nurse on duty, you know that the correct development is:

a. At 4 weeks the baby is 0.4cm, 0.4 g

b. At 4 weeks the baby is 4cm, 4g

c. At 4 weeks the baby is 0.3cm, 0.3g

d. At 4 weeks the baby is 4.3cm, 4g

39. A pregnant woman in her 8th month has been gaining weight and her husband is concerned that her wife is eating too much. The woman always reasons that two of them are eating. The nurse attending to the couple in the family clinic addresses this problem by saying that the total weight gain during pregnancy should be:

   a. 10-20lbs
   b. 15-25lbs
   c. 20-30lbs
   d. 25-35lbs

40. A mother brought her child to the ER department after seeing that her child accidentally swallowed acetaminophen. The child is only 6 years old, and the mother doesn't know how many tablets the child drank. All she knows is that the bottle is half full, but now nearly gone. Which of the following should the nurse do first?

   a. Gastric lavage
   b. Administer acetylcysteine
   c. Start IVF
   d. Administer activated charcoal

41. Mr. Pon underwent cardiac catheterization and was brought back to his room. As the nurse in charge of taking care of him, what should you monitor for the first 24 hours after the procedure?

   a. Chest pain, even at rest
   b. Signs and symptoms of thrombus formation
   c. Dizziness
   d. Decrease or falling blood pressure

42. You are a volunteer in a medical mission in a rural area. Most of the patients are senior citizens. You are checking the blood pressure of one patient and you got 160/90 mmHg. The patient told you that his BP is usually not that high. What would your response be?

   a. Tell the patient to have her BP checked within 2-3 days.

b. Tell him to seek medical help, or consult his doctor.

c. Tell him that he's just probably tired.

d. Tell him that his BP is normal as it is not in the hospital.

43. A surprised disaster drill was sounded off during the evening shift. As the charge nurse on the medical ward, which of the following patients will you list first for discharge to have rooms to the new admissions?

 a. 43-year old male, with a history of being dependent on a ventilator for 4 years, hospitalized for 4 days due to pneumonia.

 b. 24-year old female suffering from Diabetes Mellitus, Type 2 for 5 years, admitted due to vomiting and diarrhea a day ago.

 c. A 55-year old male with history of chronic heart disease, admitted due to hypertension and inability to swallow food.

 d. A 31-year old male with pneumonia for 5 days admitted due to fever and cellulitis of the lower leg 2 days ago.

44. In a consultation unit, the physician prescribed Levothyroxine to the patient for her hypothyroidism. The client asks the clinic nurse how to take the medication. The best response would be:

 a. "It should be taken in the morning after breakfast."

 b. "You must take it 30 minutes to one hour before breakfast."

 c. "You can dissolve it in juice or water to help you ingest it."

 d. "You can take it together with your other medications."

45. The nurse is discussing with the parents about diabetes mellitus in school age children. Which of the following signs is important for parents to have their child be evaluated?

 a. Increased preference to sweet food

 b. Increased intake of fluids

 c. Bed wetting

 d. Sudden decrease in weight

46. A man is worried about the pregnancy of his wife, as he wants his baby and his wife to be healthy, but not obese. He told you that his sisters were so big when they got pregnant and had difficulty giving birth. He asks Nurse Pam what is the additional caloric intake for his wife. What is the correct response?

    a. "She needs an additional 300cal per day."

    b. "She just needs to continue with her regular diet."

    c. "Make sure she has 500cal per day added."

    d. "It's okay to eat whatever she likes."

47. A female model went for consultation about her pelvic inflammatory disease. As the nurse, you are knowledgeable that this disease results from what infection?

    a. Streptococcus

    b. Chlamydia

    c. Trichomoniasis

    d. Staphylococcus

48. A coronary heart disease patient is ready for discharge. The following should be included in the nurse health teachings, EXCEPT:

    a. Light to moderate exercise such as walking.

    b. Avoiding heavy meals.

    c. Limit sodium intake to 7g in a day.

    d. Eating 3 balanced meals in a day.

49. During one of the nurses' rounds, Nurse Mae is alerted that one of her patients, post left CVA, is weakening. Which of the following caused her to think that way?

    a. Decreased level of consciousness

    b. Altered eating pattern

    c. Altered sensation to stimuli

    d. Decreased emotional stability

50. Your patient, Rica, is for radiography exam of her Kidney, Ureter, and Bladder (KUB). What should you instruct her to do prior to the procedure?

    a. The night before, ask her to no longer ingest anything (NPO).

    b. 2 hours before the procedure she will undergo enema.

    c. Ask her to take a bath before the procedure.

    d. There is nothing to instruct her, as no special preparation is needed.

51. A patient in the labor room is complaining of abdominal pain and tells the nurse that her baby is coming out. Upon assessment, the nurse is sure that the patient is a candidate for cesarian section because of EXCEPT:

    a. The passenger is in a breech presentation.

    b. The passageway is not opening.

    c. The power of contractions is not continuous and relieved by walking.

    d. The patient's anxiety is heightened causing irregular FHT.

52. A mother is concerned that her 3-year old child is playful and naughty. She said that she always reprove him every time. And this causes her child to grouch at times. The nurse understands that the child is on what stage?

    a. Industry vs. Inferiority

    b. Trust vs. Mistrust

    c. Initiative vs. Guilt

    d. Autonomy vs. Shame and Doubt

53. The staff nurse is observing the student nurse on how she feeds a patient via nasogastric tube. The staff nurse knows that everything the student nurse is doing is correct, EXCEPT:

    a. Verify the correct placement of the tube.

    b. Position the patient in a semi to high fowler's position.

    c. Aspirate the contents and flush with water if content is 200ml and below.

    d. Ensure that the solution is at room temperature.

54. Nurse Cathy is caring for a patient on a cardiac monitor and an IV line of 20mEq KCL in 500ml of D5W. Previous lab results show that the patient has a 3.2mEq/L level of Potassium. Cathy knows that if the EKG monitor shows this, the infusion needs to be stopped.

    a. Prominent 'U' waves

    b. 'ST' segment shortening

    c. Peaked 'T' wave

    d. Prolonged 'QT'

55. A child was brought to the emergency department because of the following symptoms: a painless lump on the neck, nose bleeding, and tingling/numbness and loss of movement. The nurse suspected that this is a common cancer found in children, which is:

    a. Acute Lymphocytic Leukemia

    b. Neuroblastoma

    c. Rhabdomyosarcoma

    d. CNS tumors

56. A patient in the delivery room is assessed by the attending physician. According to the assessment, the patient has 2 cms dilatation, with full effacement! As the nurse, you know that the patient is on what kind of phase and stage?

    a. Stage I, active phase.

    b. Stage I, latent phase.

    c. Stage II, transition phase.

    d. Stage II, active phase.

57. The nurse is knowledgeable about the difference of false labor with true labor. The following are symptoms of labor, which pair is for false labor:

I. Intensity of contraction is progressive and increases with walking.

II. Contractions are inconsistent in pattern.

III. The discomfort felt on abdomen and groin.

IV. Durations of contractions vary.

   b. I, II, III

   c. II, III, IV

   d. I, III, IV

   e. II, IV, I

58. A nurse in the pediatric ward should be aware that a 1-year old patient with this symptom should be reported immediately:

   a. Rapid breathing followed by shallow breathing.

   b. Abdominal Breathing.

   c. Inspiratory grunts or gurgles.

   d. Frequent sneezing.

59. A patient with a healing venous stasis ulcer is ready for discharge. As part of the nurse's discharge instruction is to promote continuous healing of the ulcer. Which of the following should be included in the plan of care?

   a. Proper wound dressing and cleaning techniques.

   b. Elevation of the leg when sleeping.

   c. Plan for debridement of wound on the next consultation.

   d. Improve the patient's nutritional status.

60. A patient with multiple sclerosis is wondering if she is allowed to exercise. The nurse, after explaining the importance, tells the client, "It is okay to exercise as long as…"

   a. …you monitor your heart rate."

   b. …you increase your fluid intake."

c. ...you choose the aerobic program."

d. ...you become involved in competitive sports."

61. In the clinic, while waiting for his turn to see the doctor, one patient approaches the nurse and asks about his nutritional diet. Checking his records reveal that he has Addison's disease. Which is the best response of the nurse?

   a. "You should have high caloric intake."

   b. "You should decrease protein intake."

   c. "Grains are not your friend."

   d. "You should limit sodium intake."

62. A diabetic patient underwent cholecystectomy and is now in the second day post-operative period. She is currently on a diet as tolerated, however, her relatives told the nurse that she is unable to eat or drink. The nurse observes that the patient is confused and shaky. Which of the following exhibits the patient's condition?

   a. There is still anesthesia left in her body.

   b. She is full and suffering from hyperglycemia.

   c. She has hypoglycemia.

   d. This is a case of diabetic ketoacidosis.

63. A patient underwent fiberoptic colonoscopy for as part of their company's annual physical examination. The nurse teaching the patient on the possible complications of the procedure is talking about bowel perforation. The symptoms include:

   a. Abdominal pain, fever, chills and tachycardia.

   b. Abdominal pain, bleeding, chills, and fever.

   c. Bleeding, mass in the abdomen, abdominal pain and fever.

   d. Decrease in the size of abdomen, fever, chills and tachycardia.

64. In the ward, two patients are talking about their medications. Patient A has rheumatoid arthritis and patient B has acute gastritis. Patient A says that he takes two medications at once, naproxen sodium and antacid. Patient B says, "Perhaps, I can also take naproxen sodium." The nurse overhearing their conversation approaches them to:

    a. Tell them they are being noisy, other patients are resting.

    b. Join their conversation and talk about their different medications.

    c. Explain to them the reason of taking the medications.

    d. Stop patient B from taking the medication of patient A.

65. A hospitalized patient in the cardiac unit was suddenly transferred to the intensive care because of air hunger. The ICU nurse knows that this is a symptom of:

    a. Myocardial infarction

    b. Laryngeal Swelling

    c. Pulmonary edema

    d. Cardiac shock

66. A nurse is giving lectures on pregnancy, the nutritional intake, weight gain, development of the fetus, and many more. One pregnant woman asks the nurse about gestational diabetes. What should the nurse respond on the question, "Will I also need to inject insulin?"

    a. "Insulin is the basic treatment for diabetes."

    b. "Insulin should only be a last resort for gestational diabetes."

    c. "Yes, you will, and it will be for a lifetime."

    d. "No, there are oral antidiabetic drugs if you can't inject insulin."

67. During shift endorsement, the charge nurse is reading the different procedures the patients in the ward will be undergoing at 8am. As an incoming nurse, and in charge of the left wing, you heard that one of your patients will undergo an implantable cardioverter defibrillator. Which of the following will undergo the procedure?

    a. Patient A with irregular ECG result on nitroglycerin.

b. Patient B with a history of atrial tachycardia, admitted due to fatigue.

c. Patient C with a history of ventricular tachycardia with syncope.

d. Patient D with bradycardia and hypotension.

68. A nurse is preparing a patient for an MRI, diagnostic procedure to inspect for possible liver cancer. Which of the following is a contraindication to diagnostic exam?

    a. Allergy to shellfish or iodine.

    b. Having an implanted pacemaker.

    c. Fear of tight spaces.

    d. The patient has heart medications.

69. A patient was rushed to the ER department with complaints of abdominal pain, radiating to the back. Work-ups reveal that the patient has a rapidly enlarging abdominal aortic aneurysm. What should the nurse expect to be the next action?

    a. Admission of the patient to the medical ward with close monitoring.

    b. Admission of the patient to the medical ward for medication and close monitoring.

    c. Admission of the patient to the surgical ward and scheduling of resection.

    d. Admission of the patient to the surgical ward for scheduling of Sclerotherapy.

70. A patient with leukemia suddenly became pale after chemotherapy. The physician ordered to check for blood count as the next step. It revealed a platelet count of 20,000/microliter. What should be the next action of the nurse?

    a. Limit visitors as the patient is prone to infection.

    b. Ask every visitor to perform handwashing, wear mask and gloves.

    c. Anticipate cross matching of PRBC.

    d. Monitor for signs of bleeding.

71. In the pediatric unit of the ER department, the doctor is assessing a child with scarlet fever. The nurse knows that the signs and symptoms of the disease includes the following, EXCEPT:

    a. "Strawberry tongue"

    b. Red lines found in the folds of the body.

    c. Petechiae on the soft palate.

    d. Swollen neck glands.

72. A nurse in the maternal ward is continually monitoring a patient with placenta previa. The patient is on bed rest and fetal monitoring is attached to her abdomen. Suddenly, the patient asks for help as she felt fluid coming out of her. The nurse knows that the complication of placenta previa is:

    a. Rupture of placenta.

    b. Suffocation of the baby.

    c. Hypovolemic shock.

    d. Blood dyscrasia.

73. A 23-year old student was admitted due to the difficulty of urination and fever. She has a history of recurring urinary tract infection. The doctor suspects that this time it is acute glomerulonephritis. Lab results will reveal the following, EXCEPT:

    a. Physical appearance: brown

    b. Specific Gravity: 1.040

    c. Protein: present

    d. Glucose: negative

74. In the newborn care unit, a mother approaches the nurse about her son. "I think there is water in the scrotum of my child." The best response by the nurse would be:

    a. "I will notify the doctor right away."

    b. "You must massage the scrotum of your child."

    c. "There is nothing wrong with your child."

d. "There is no need to worry as fluid in the scrotum at his age is normal."

75. A patient with peripheral vascular disease (PVD) experiences pain in her leg muscles. This is due to the increased demand of oxygen, but lesser supply. This pain is known as:

a. Arthralgia

b. Breakthrough pain

c. Claudication

d. Neuropathic pain

76. A 36-year old pregnant woman, multipara, tells the clinic nurse that she is not expecting this pregnancy. She feels that something will go wrong, and it is risky for her and for her baby. However, she also told the nurse that she has no intention of aborting the pregnancy. The nurse knows that the main concern for her case is:

a. Placenta previa

b. Pre-eclampsia

c. Gestational Diabetes

d. Placenta Abruptio

77. A patient with a history of stroke was in a clinic for a follow-up. During the initial assessment, the nurse checked his vitals and his compliance with medications. The patient showed one of his medications and asked the nurse for its action. What should the nurse say about thrombolytic therapy?

I. It's taken to break down lipids in the body.

II. The most common example is tPAs.

III. Cerebral hemorrhage is a complication.

a. I and II

b. II and III

c. I and III

d. All of the above

78. At a conference, a nurse Amy is showing to the student nurses how to assess a certain disease. She asks for a volunteer to stand in front. She told the student nurse to face the front (that way her back is showing at the audience), and to bend forward at her waist and her hands dangling freely. Nurse Amy asks the students what disease is being assessed.

    a. Balance and coordination

    b. Orthostatic hypotension

    c. Spinal flexibility

    d. Scoliosis

79. At a school clinic, the clinic nurse is interviewing a mother about her child. Her child is not performing well in school, timid, and at times aloof. The mother started crying, keeps blaming herself, and repeatedly saying that she is a single mother. The nurse knows that these are characteristics of:

    a. Psychosis

    b. Abusive parent

    c. Poor family

    d. Low self-esteem

80. A mother of a child with juvenile idiopathic arthritis is asking the nurse on the treatment and long term effect of the disease to her child. The nurse knows that the mother was able to understand the explanation if:

    a. "The disease will affect him until he becomes an adult."

    b. "I need to give him pain medication for 3-4 weeks."

    c. "He should not join any sports activity anymore."

    d. "Physically, his joints will be deformed."

81. Mrs. Tan shows her concern as her child was diagnosed to have cerebral palsy. To lessen her worries in taking care of her child and increase her knowledge about the disease, the nurse discussed the following. Which of them is NOT a correct information about cerebral palsy?

    a. Mrs. Tan needs to bring her child for a regular developmental screening, this will prevent secondary delays.

    b. The disease affects the upper motor neurons. The child will likely have motor dysfunction, visual and speech problems.

    c. The child's development is slightly delayed, but doesn't need any intervention.

    d. Sharing with a support group will help Mrs. Tan.

82. During the night shift, a patient with frostbite is rushed to the emergency department. His feet are immediately soaked in hot water for rapid continuous rewarming. The purpose of the intervention is:

    a. To encourage blood flow in the area affected.

    b. To decrease the amount of damage to cells and tissues.

    c. To alleviate pain felt in the affected area.

    d. To make the patient warm since he came from a cold area.

83. A newly diagnosed ESRD patient is afraid to undergo dialysis. Nurse Max knows the need to educate the patient. He knows that dialysis is important, because:

    a. It decreases blood pressure and replaces the body with new blood.

    b. It allows you to eat all the food you enjoy because it will clean your body.

    c. It keeps the body functioning normally by filtering toxic waste from the blood.

    d. It is fast, easy, convenient and will not cause any pain.

84. A pregnant woman in 25wks AOG, was brought to the ER department due to headache, and visual disturbances. Her BP was taken and is 160/90mmHg. The nurse knows that these are symptoms of:

    a. Seizure

b. Premature labor

c. Pre-eclampsia

d. Hyperemesis gravidarum

85. A community nurse is going to visit her patient who has a diagnosis of AIDS. During the interview, the patient said that he didn't know his nephew who came to visit him yesterday has measles. The nurse knows that the next action to be done is:

a. Perform cleaning of the house to remove any bacteria.

b. Notify the physician for immunoglobulin.

c. Be strict in limiting visitors of the patient.

d. Advise the patient to take his antibiotic immediately.

86. The nurse doing her rounds entered the room of a client who undergone above-the-knee amputation. The patient told the nurse that he feels pain in his foot. Which is the best response of the nurse to the patient experiencing phantom limb pain?

a. "Just do deep breathing exercises and the pain will go away."

b. "I will get you some pain medications right away."

c. "Let's use guided imagery, because you no longer have a foot."

d. "Let us check your leg, perhaps which is the part painful."

87. During the first trimester of her pregnancy, Claire experienced nausea and vomiting in different hours of the day. It interrupts her work and it worries her. Her husband says, "Isn't that a normal thing?" Nurse Cath knows that Claire:

a. Is exaggerating her pregnancy, and should not be entertained.

b. Is experiencing a high emotional instability, therefore, should be admitted.

c. Is experiencing a vomiting disorder for pregnant women.

d. Is stressed and is affecting her pregnancy.

88. A patient with pancreatic cancer asked the nurse, "The doctor said I have to undergo Whipple procedure, will they totally remove my pancreas?" The nurse knows that Whipple procedure is:

a. To remove only the head of the pancreas.

b. To remove the pancreas and the proximal part of the small intestines.

c. To remove the half of the pancreas.

d. To remove the affected part of the pancreas and affected nearby organs.

89. Nurse Pam is assisting in the doctor's removal of a central venous catheter. She instructs the patient to bear down and hold her breath. This is important because:

a. It elevates the venous pressure above the atmospheric pressure.

b. It makes it less likely for air to enter the venous system.

c. It will prevent blood loss and air entry.

d. It will allow air to be aspirated into the systemic circulation.

90. The doctor has a new order of streptokinase for the patient of Nurse Ji. Which of the following will make Nurse Ji question the doctor's order?

a. Allergies to sea shells and seafood.

b. History of seizures and intake of phenytoin.

c. History of streptococcal infections.

d. History of alcohol addiction.

91. Lydia is pregnant with her second child. She tells the nurse that when lying flat in bed she feels dizzy, at times nauseatic, and feels her heart beating fast. The nurse knows that she is experiencing Supine Hypotensive Syndrome. The best action for the nurse is:

a. To encourage patient to sleep in a semi-fowler's position.

b. Teach deep breathing exercises to increase oxygen supply.

c. To position the patient on the left side when lying down.

d. To reassure the patient that medications will be given.

92. In changing the tracheostomy ties, without an assistant, the nurse should first prepare all the things at the bedside. She should also prepare herself such as hand washing and donning gloves. And she should be aware that it is best to:

   a. Place the new tracheostomy tie first before removing the old one.

   b. Support the tracheostomy tube with the dominant hand.

   c. Support the tracheostomy with the non-dominant hand while the dominant hand will cut the old ties.

   d. Let the surgeon perform the task, you are not qualified to do it.

93. A patient with pneumothorax due to a vehicular accident now has a chest tube in place. The nurse checking for the hourly output of the drain saw 250ml output. What is the best action of the nurse?

   a. Change the position of the patient, from one side to the other.

   b. Check for the patency of the chest tube.

   c. Decrease the IV Infusion.

   d. Notify the physician.

94. A student nurse has a task of monitoring a patient with a case of Tetralogy of Fallot. The nurse on duty asked the student nurse what are the diseases included in tetralogy of Fallot. The student nurse is correct in saying the following, EXCEPT:

   a. Ventral Septal Defect

   b. Pulmonary Stenosis

   c. Overriding Aorta

   d. Aortic Valve Stenosis

95. In question #94, which is the best drug of choice for the patient?

   a. Digoxin

   b. Epinephrine

   c. Aminophylline

   d. Atropine

96. A G2P1, in her 20weeks AOG, but had a stillbirth, is concerned that her pregnancy will result in that way again. As the nurse, you explained the importance of the nonstress test. This is to:

    a. Verify the maturity of the fetal lung.

    b. Assess and gauge fetal activity.

    c. Determine the fetal heart rate.

    d. Check the quantity of the amniotic fluid.

97. The nurse is assisting a pregnant patient with prolapsed cord. The nurse knows that things to ensure the safety of the fetus, the cord and the baby is:

    a. Cover the cord with saline-soaked gauze.

    b. Push the cord back into the uterus.

    c. Encourage mother to bear down.

    d. Place patient in trendelenburg if birth is imminent.

98. An office clerk resigned from her work because of recurrence of UTI. She told the nurse that the comfort room is not clean that is why she always get the infection. The nurse knows that the probable cause of her UTI is due to:

    a. Continence or holding of urine

    b. Wiping from front to back after urinating.

    c. Drinking acidic and citrus fluids.

    d. Having 8-10 glasses of water daily.

99. The nurse in the ward has to multitask in order to complete the necessary plan of care for her shift. She is aided by a nursing assistant. Among the following patients, what activity should be given to the assistant:

    a. Assisting in the ambulation of a patient with a fractured hip.

    b. Checking the IFC output of a pregnant patient with pre-eclampsia.

    c. Placing a tuberculosis patient in isolation.

    d. Providing food and feeding the patient with dementia.

100. The nurse is receiving a patient from the operating room with a case of post-op thyroidectomy. What should equipment should the nurse place on standby at the patient's bedside?

    a. An endotracheal tube

    b. A bag-mask valve

    c. A tracheostomy set

    d. A padded tongue depressor

ANSWERS:

1. Correct Answer: C.

The patient on oxygen therapy, mostly need rest, do not let her sit, instead elevate the head part of the bed and let her do DBE to increase oxygen intake. The coughing exercises will loosen any secretions. You must not just increase the oxygen administration, but titrate it in order to attain an SPO2 of 95%. These make choices A, B and D incorrect.

2. Correct Answer: D.

Diabetes is a disease that does not concern the exchange of oxygen, the amount of oxygen needed, or transport of oxygen to different parts of the body, which are exhibited by choices A, B, and C.

3. Correct Answer: A.

If there are no problems with the ventilator nor the ET tube, then it is not recommended to change them, making choices B wrong. Note that the condition of the patient is difficult to ventilate, restless and has shown ineffective ventilation. Do not reposition the patient, nor use BVM to ventilate. The choice is to sedate the patient to relax him and promote more exchange of oxygen.

4. Correct Answer: B.

System disconnection or leaks cause Low-pressure alarm. A high-pressure alarm is due to choice C and patient biting. High-Respiratory Rate alarm is shown in choice A. And Low Exhaled Volume alarm is due to choice D.

5. Correct Answer: C.

A nurse is a trained personnel qualified to keep the tracheotomy tube open, and to care for the tube. With sterile equipment the nurse can secure the tube. An LPNs are not qualified to perform the task, BVM should only be used if the patient cannot breath. Therefore, A, B, and D are incorrect.

6. Correct Answer: C.

Continuous bubbling in the chest tube's water seal chamber means that the tube is disconnected, or breaks, incomplete seal around the tube insertion site, or the tube is not inserted properly.

7. Correct Answer: D.

This is obviously a case of the chest tube being dislodged. Remove the old dressing and cover the site with a sterile occlusive dressing immediately, before doing A, B and C.

8. Correct Answer: C.

Salem sumps have air vents and are used for suction and irrigation. A, B, and D are correct procedures in feeding a patient with NGT.

9. Correct Answer: B.

This is a sign of aspiration ad gastric reflux and is caused when there is improper placement of the tube, delayed gastric emptying or the patient was not placed in semifowler's position before, during and after feeding. It has nothing to do with the patient's history of CHD.

10. Correct Answer: A.

Choices B and C are not correct as the blood has an IVF in it. There is no need to let the patient sign unless she refuses the procedure. The best place to draw the blood sample is on the right arm.

11. Correct Answer: B.

Allen Test is a test performed to assess sufficient collateral circulation, therefore blood sample can be taken in the area. Choices A, C and D are just made up.

12. Correct Answer: B.

24 hour urine collection entails the collection of urine that usually starts between 6 and 8 am, the first void thrown away and all the subsequent urine are collected. To minimize and prevent bacterial growth, all collected should be refrigerated placed on ice, not necessarily frozen. Every bottle should be sent to the laboratory at the end of the collection.

13. Correct Answer: C.

Sputum test should be done before drinking any antimicrobial agents as this a part of the diagnostics. All the other choices are correct.

14. Correct Answer: D.

Cheyenne-Stokes indicates a neurological condition characterized by alternating patterns of depth separated by brief periods of apnea. Apneustic is also neurologic with sustained inspiratory effort. Kussmaul's is a rapid, deep and labored breathing. And Hyperventilation is rapid, deep inspiration greater an 20 breaths/minute.

15. Correct Answer: C.

Inspect the appearance of the skin. Auscultate for bowel sounds. Percuss for abdominal tone. And Palpate any pulsations, masses, tenderness, and rigidity.

16. Correct Answer: D.

Deep Vein Thrombosis has the following signs and symptoms: Homans' sign (calf pain on dorsiflexion), pain, venous distention, and localized tenderness.

17. Correct Answer: B.

Cracking in the area, also known as crepitance is an early sign of gangrene. The physician should be notified immediately when this happens.

18. Correct Answer: C.

Stage V is considered as the stage of pressure ulcer covered with eschar and cannot be staged without debridement. Stage I indicates an erythematous area. Stage II presents as an abrasion, blister, or a very shallow crater. Stage III has a full thickness crater involving damage and/or necrosis down to, but not penetrating. Stage IV is a full thickness ulcer, similar to Stage III, but penetrating fascia with involvement of muscle and bone.

19. Correct Answer: A.

Romberg's Test. In choice B, the patient is instructed to tap the tip of thumb with tip of index finger as fast as possible. In choice C, the patient is instructed to close eyes and alternate touching index finger to the nose. In choice D, the patient is instructed to touch nose and his index finger alternately several times.

20. Correct Answer: B.

Moderate brain injury has a GCS of 9-12. Mild brain injury has a GCS of 13-14. Choices C and D are not part of the range.

21. Correct Answer: A.

The nurse will be able to reduce the patient's body temperature by decreasing the room temperature, and process of convection. Other ways include tepid sponge bath, cool compress and cooling blankets. Antipyretic can also be given, encourage fluid intake. Continuous monitoring could be done, but not every two hours.

22. Correct Answer: D.

The best nursing intervention in reducing pain to the patient that received a burn injury is to administer pain medications. Apply cool packs and not warm to reduce swelling in the area. The wound should be kept dry and clean. And elevating patient's arm does not help in reducing pain; it increases venous return to the heart.

23. Correct Answer: B.

Kegel's exercise and not Valsalva maneuver is responsible in strengthening the muscles in the perineal area. Indwelling Foley catheter increases the risk for infection. Pads or diapers should only be a last resort.

24. Correct Answer: B.

The patient will now depend on his capability to manage his health. Therefore, he must be able to adapt to his home environment in maintaining his health and how to cope up with his activities, such as work, family, and taking care of himself. Choices A, C, and D are part of choice B.

25. Correct Answer: D.

Remember that pain scale in only one assessment, other assessments should be performed to totally examine the pain of the patient. If pain felt is something can't be handled, administration of medication should not be withheld, notify the staff nurse for the pain medication of the patient.

26. Correct Answer: D.

Orange juice and banana contain potassium. Other food includes raisins, apricots, beans, avocados, and potatoes.

27. Correct Answer: C.

The total intake is 8 oz = 480ml, 950ml, 1 cup = 240ml, 800ml. Adding them 480+950+240+800 = 2,470.

28. Correct Answer: D.

The normal range of Calcium is 4.5 -5.5 mEq/L. Trousseau's sign refers to carpopedal spasm that happens after 2-5 minutes after applying and inflating the blood pressure cuff to above 20mmHg on the upper arm. Chvostek's sign is the twitching of the facial nerve.

29. Correct Answer: D.

For patients with COPD, the main stimulus is when the breathing becomes hypoxia or low PO2. A high PO2 indicates increase in O2 levels and therefore not a stimulus for breathing. High pCO2 means there is an inadequate response of the respiratory center to the plasma carbon dioxide. A Low pCO2 is not a normal finding in patients with obstructive lung disease.

30. Correct Answer: B.

The normal range for magnesium id 1.5-2.5mEq/L. Therefore the patient suffers from hypomagnesemia, which puts her at risk for injury due to seizure attacks. The nurse should perform seizure precautions. Choice A is for Hypophophatemia where there is a change in granulocytes. Choice C is for peudohyperkalemia. Choice D is not related.

31. Correct Answer: C.

Sodium and Chlorine values of the patient are within normal range. Potassium on the other hand is elevated; normal range is 3.5 – 5.5mEq/L. Therefore the nurse should anticipate a medication that will lower the K levels. Kayexalate is a cation-exchange resin that helps to reduce potassium from the intestines and excreted through the feces. Calcium gluconate is a supplement for low calcium levels and antidote for MgSO4.

32. Correct Answer: C.

Potassium level. Diuretics like furosemide does not spare potassium, therefore it is excreted through the urine. This increases the action of digoxin and the risk of digoxin toxicity. Therefore, the nurse should monitor the serum potassium levels. Choices A, B, and D are not related to the medications.

33. Correct Answer: C.

3. Gravida refers to the number of pregnancy, regardless of the outcome, including the current pregnancy.

34. Correct Answer: B.

GTPAL stands for Gravida (number of all pregnancies), Term (for all pregnancies that reach the maximum AOG), Preterm (for all pregnancies that did not reach the desired AOG), Abortion (including miscarriages), and Living (those that are alive at birth).

35. Correct Answer: C.

LGA stands for Large for Gestational Age which means that the baby's birth weight is greater than the 90th percentile or greater than 4000g. Other choices are not related to LGA.

36. Correct Answer: D.

Organogenesis starts from week 3 to week 8.

37. Correct Answer: B.

Nagele's Rule: Add 7 days to the first day of LMP. Subtract 3 months. Add one year. LMP: May 20, 2015 = 05/20/2015 (add 7 days) = 05/27/2015 (subtract 3 months) = 02/27/2015 (add one year) = 02/27/2016.

38. Correct Answer: A.

According to the Fetal Development Timetable, at 4 weeks the baby is 0.4cm, 0.4g

39. Correct Answer: D.

25-35lbs is the total weight gain during pregnancy. Too much glucose and carbohydrates will have some side effects in pregnancy and to the baby.

40. Correct Answer: A.

Gastric lavage should be the priority of the nurse to remove as much of the ingested drug as possible. It can be followed by administering activated charcoal, acetylcysteine, then the IVF.

41. Correct Answer: B.

After cardiac catheterization, a potential problem is the formation of thrombus in the coronary artery. This can happen in the first 24 hours after the procedure. S/S includes shortness of breath, sharp/stabbing chest pain, and fast heart rate. Dizziness and falling blood pressure are signs of hemorrhage at the insertion site.

42. Correct Answer: A.

If the blood pressure reading is moderately high; there is the need to have it rechecked within 2-3 days or 48-72 hours. The nurse should also assess possible underlying cause of the increase in the patient's blood pressure making choice C incorrect. Choices B and D as it gives a warning to the patient.

43. Correct Answer: A.

The perfect candidate for discharge is a patient who has the ability to continue care at home. The choice A shows that the patient had a chronic disease before and is familiar with his case now. He is the most stable among the patients presented.

44. Correct Answer: B.

Levothyroxine is taken in a single dose daily, preferably 30 minutes to one hour before breakfast. It should be taken at least 4 hours before taking other medications. It should be swallowed whole and should be crushed or dissolved in liquids.

45. Correct Answer: C.

School age children no longer wet during their sleep. However, for children with a possible diagnosis of diabetes mellitus, bed wetting and fatigue are two observable conditions that should prompt the parents to seek medical evaluation.

46. Correct Answer: A.

The additional caloric requirement of a pregnant woman is 300 cal/day. This is broken down to: protein -75g, carb -175g (mostly complex), fiber -28g, fats - 20-35g, fluid -3L/day (unless pre-eclampsia exist), iron -27mg, calcium -1000mg, folic acid -6000mcg.

47. Correct Answer: B.

Chlamydia affects the genitourinary tract and is the common cause of PID and salpingitis.

48. Correct Answer: C.

Limiting sodium intake to 7g in a day is necessary if the physician ordered. However, it is not necessary as long as fluid intake is sufficient.

49. Correct Answer: A.

Decreased level of consciousness is the best indicator of a patient's condition. Choices B, C, and D needs to be observed longer and are not the best indicator of progression of CVA.

50. Correct Answer: D.

KUB is one of the procedures that do not entail any special procedures, except that the patient needs to bring a liter of drinking water. Although it is a good practice to take a bath, it is not necessary for the procedure. A female patient can douche her perineal area before the procedure.

51. Correct Answer: C.

Passenger, Passageway, Power and Psychological are the 4Ps affecting the progression of labor. Choices A, B and D are factors that affect the delivery if it would be cesarean section. Choice C indicates a sign of false labor.

52. Correct Answer: D.

Children from 1 ½ to 3 years want to explore their surroundings and do things on their own. However, when stopped by an authority (in this case the mother) he will show shame and doubt.

53. Correct Answer: C.

The contents should be less than 150ml and flushed with 20ml of water. If greater than 150 to 200ml, the amount should be deducted from the feeding solution. If greater than 200ml, withhold the feeding and check after 4 hours.

54. Correct Answer: C.

Tall or peaked 'T' waves signify Hyperkalemia. Choice A is for Hypokalemia. Choice B is Hypercalcemia. And choice D is Hypocalcemia.

55. Correct Answer: C.

Rhabdomyosarcoma affects all the striated muscles in the body and is characterized by painless lump, bleeding of the nose, genitals, or where the lump is, tingling/numbness and loss of movement, and protrusion of the eyes.

56. Correct Answer: B.

Stage I, latent phase. Stage II has no phases. Stage I has three phases depending on the dilation – 0-3cms for latent, 4-7cms for active, and 8-10cms for transition.

57. Correct Answer: B.

False labor has inconsistent or varying patterns of contractions with no significant changes in the effacement and discomfort is mostly abdominal and groin.

58. Correct Answer: C.

Inspiratory grunts and gurgles are symptoms of respiratory distress and should be reported to the physician immediately. Choice A shows periodic breathing, which they will eventually outgrow. Choice B and D are normal.

59. Correct Answer: D.

Healing can occur with the right diet for the patient, therefore reinforcing it even for home care is vital. A and B are also important, but should be aided with proper nutrition. Choice C is a doctor's recommendation only.

60. Correct Answer: B.

Dehydration and/or not drinking enough fluids are among of the causes of Multiple Sclerosis. This could lead to worsening of the symptoms felt. Exercise is recommended as long as the physician is notified of the type of exercise you are into.

61. Correct Answer: D.

A patient with Addison's disease does not need to limit sodium intake. In fact, it needs a normal dietary intake of sodium in order to prevent fluid loss.

62. Correct Answer: C.

Looking at her condition, she was unable to eat and became confused and shaky. This is a symptom of hypoglycemia, as the patient's body is going through too much stress without enough glucose in the body.

63. Correct Answer: A.

Bowel perforation means that a hole was created due to the procedure. The symptoms include abdominal pain, fever, chills and tachycardia.

64. Correct Answer: C.

The nurse should explain to patient B that Naproxen Sodium is contraindicated in her case. Merely stopping her without explanation will not get her cooperation.

65. Correct Answer: C.

A patient suffering from pulmonary edema exhibits: air hunger, agitation, anxiety, and tachycardia.

66. Correct Answer: B.

Pregnant women who developed Diabetes are not recommended to have insulin injections immediately. Dietary modifications and exercise program are prescribed to help alleviate the situation and also control the complications of pregnancy such as neonatal hypoglycemia and macrosomia. Insulin should only be started if dietary management fails.

67. Correct Answer: C.

The indication for ICD (Implantable Cardioverter Defibrillator) are the following: history or an episode of ventricular tachycardia or ventricular fibrillation; previous cardiac arrest; conditions wherein the medication is no longer effective.

68. Correct Answer: B.

MRI stands for magnetic resonance imaging, which means it uses magnetic fields to scan the patient's body. This will interfere with the patient's pace maker. The contrast used is not iodine based, making choice A wrong. Choice C can be alleviated by anti-anxiety medications or with the use of open MRI. Choice D has nothing to do with MRI.

69. Correct Answer: C.

A rapidly enlarging abdominal aortic aneurysm is at risk of rupture and will cause hemorrhage if not resected the closest time possible. There are no other options when it comes to treatment, even medications can't prevent rupture.

70. Correct Answer: D.

The normal platelet count is 150,000 to 400,000. Less than that amount is considered thrombocytopenic. However, bleeding occurs when the platelet count drops to 10,000 to 20,000 per microliter.

71. Correct Answer: C.

Here are the signs and symptoms of scarlet fever: Rash (starts on the chest and stomach, sand-like texture), Swollen neck glands (such as the pharynx), Nausea and vomiting, Red lines found in the folds of the body (ex. Armpit), and Strawberry tongue (red-swollen tongue with white coating).

72. Correct Answer: C.

Pregnant women diagnosed with placenta previa is monitored for bleeding, maternal vital signs as well as fetal movement and heart rate (to check for fetal distress). Bleeding is a sign of hypovolemic shock and shows danger for the mother and her child.

73. Correct Answer: D.

Urinalysis for the patient is very important as it will reveal the presence of protein, RBCs, WBCs, casts and fats in the urine. The specific gravity is rather high, the normal range is 1.010 – 1.030, and it presents a darker colored urine.

74. Correct Answer: D.

A baby, in this case, exhibits hydrocele. However, there is no need for any intervention as the fluid will be reabsorbed in the first few months of the child.

75. Correct Answer: C.

Claudication is characterized by leg pain and weakness upon walking, and loss of pain when rested. Breakthrough pain is an acute pain managed with medication. Arthralgia is joint pain. And Neuropathic pain is due to damage to a part of the nervous system.

76. Correct Answer: D.

Placenta Abruptio affects multiparous women, ages 35 and up, with no known cause, but is associated with pre-eclampsia and HTN. Choice B is characterized by HTN. Choice C is development of diabetes during pregnancy. And choice A refers to a condition where the placenta is in the lower segment of the uterus.

77. Correct Answer: B.

The most common drug given to stroke patients undergoing thrombolytic therapy is tPAs, which stands for tissue plasminogen activator. Its main action is to break down blood clots.

In long term therapy, the patient must be monitored for signs of bleeding, especially cerebral hemorrhage.

78. Correct Answer: D.

Scoliosis is a deviation of the spine. With the position of the volunteer, it would be easier to check any curvature (lateral) and/or rib deformities.

79. Correct Answer: B.

The activities that the parents do to their child reflects on how the child is doing at school. In this case the single mother presents the signs of her being abusive. These are low self-esteem, single status and self-blame of what happened to her child.

80. Correct Answer: B.

Pain medications are given to relieve the pain felt, NSAIDs is the drug of choice. It will not progress to adult rheumatoid arthritis, or joint deformities. Physical activity is part of the therapeutic regimen.

81. Correct Answer: C.

Regular screening is needed to help the child cope up with the delayed developmental milestones. The child's difficulties should have interventions such as therapies.

82. Correct Answer: B.

This intervention is designed to lessen the damage to the cells and tissues caused by frostbite. It might cause pain, but a good signal that feeling is coming back to the area.

83. Correct Answer: C.

Dialysis removes the waste and chemicals in the blood by having a catheter inserted in the arm or neck of the patient. The machine will act as an artificial kidney, since the kidney is no longer functioning.

84. Correct Answer: C.

Pre-eclampsia has an onset of 20wks AOG, mostly affects pregnant adolescents and ages 35 up. The symptoms are hypertension, edema, proteinuria, hyperreflexia, clonus, headache, visual disturbances, vasospasm, and seizures.

85. Correct Answer: B.

An AIDS patient is an immunocompromised patient. Therefore, cleaning the house, isolation and antibiotic will not do any good for the patient. The best action is to boost his immune system, therefore immunoglobulin from the physician is needed.

86. Correct Answer: B.

Phantom limb pain (PLP) is caused by the loss of sensory input from the foot, interrupting the nerve signals. This pain felt can last from several months to years. It is best to address the pain felt with the use of pain medications, as the pain felt is true for the patient and cannot be considered psychological.

87. Correct Answer: C.

What the patient is experiencing is Hyperemesis Gravidarum, or intractable nausea and vomiting during the first trimester. The feeling of wanting to vomit is normal, however, it becomes a disease when it happens anytime of the day and affects her normal activities.

88. Correct Answer: A.

The Whipple procedure is also known as pancreatoduodenectomy, is to remove the head of the pancreas, the first part of the small intestine or the duodenum, the gall bladder and a portion of the stomach. The tumor cells mostly develop in the head of the pancreas therefore, that is the only part of the pancreas to be removed.

89. Correct Answer: B.

Bearing down and holding breath is called Valsalva maneuver and is important during removal of central venous catheter to prevent air from entering the venous system. Choice A happens when the patient is in Trendelenburg position. Choice C is the rationale for applying gentle pressure the exit site of the catheter. Choice D is ensuring hydration of the patient.

90. Correct Answer: C.

Previous streptococcal infection will hinder the effectiveness of streptokinase. Choices A, B and D have no relation with the medication.

91. Correct Answer: C.

Supine Hypotensive Syndrome happens when the uterus compresses the IVC. This result to the pooling of blood in the legs, decreased venous return, decrease CO and hypotension. It will be relieved by positioning the patient in a left lateral position to remove the pressure on the IVC.

92. Correct Answer: A.

If without an assistant, the nurse should place the new tie first before removing the old ones in order to secure the tracheostomy in place and prevent it from being coughed out by the patient. The nurse is qualified to perform the action, and can do it without doctor's orders.

93. Correct Answer: D.

The normal output should be less than 5ml/kg/hour. Therefore a 250ml output for an hour is a sign of bleeding and the doctor should be notified immediately. Choice A and C will not help the patient. Choice B is not needed as there is an output, therefore it is patent.

94. Correct Answer: D.

Tetralogy of Fallot is a condition with four problems: Choice A, B, C and Right Ventricular Hypertrophy. Therefore choice D is not included.

95. Correct Answer: A.

Digoxin is the best drug of choice, as it will slow the beating of the heart and strengthen the heart contractions. Choices B, C, and D will increase the contractions, therefore overworking the heart.

96. Correct Answer: B.

The nonstress test is done to determine the periodic fetal movements. Other tests are used to determine choice A, C, and D.

97. Correct Answer: A.

Cover the cords with saline-soaked gauze to maintain cord's integrity and monitor cord pulses. Choice B and C should not be done. And only the put patient in trendelenburg if a birth is not imminent.

98. Correct Answer: A.

As an office clerk, her work entails sitting for long periods of time, at might not have the time to urinate. Choice B and D are correct practices. Choice C is still not proven to affect the occurrence of UTI.

99. Correct Answer: D.

The only activity that the nursing assistant can do is feeding the patient. The nurse or the physician is qualified to do choice A, B and D.

100. Correct Answer: C.

The tracheostomy set is needed in case the patient suffers from tracheal edema. This will help in maintaining the airway of the patient. An endotracheal tube and BVM will not help in providing ventilation to the patient. A tongue depressor is used for seizure patients.

II. NCLEX Exam Two

QUESTIONS:

1. The nurse is caring for a postpartum patient. The nurse encourages the mother to breastfeed her child. The nurse knows that breastfeeding does, EXCEPT:

   a. Prevent postpartum hemorrhage.

   b. Promotes mother-child bonding.

   c. Relieves the pain caused by childbirth.

   d. Provide the best nutrition for the baby.

2. A nurse is taking care of an elderly patient with a new physician's order of histoplasmosis test. The nurse knows that this disease is due to:

   a. Dogs

   b. Turtles

c. Birds

d. Cats

3. The nurse knows that a patient with abdominal aortic aneurysm exhibits abdominal pain. Which of the following alerts the nurse that there is an impending rupture?

a. Chest pain

b. Lower back pain

c. Left side paraplegia

d. Loss of consciousness

4. The nurse is caring for an adult patient with cardiomyopathy. Upon checking his vital signs, what is an indication of a good cardiac output?

a. Heart rate of 89.

b. BP of 150/90mmHg.

c. RR of 19.

d. Temperature of 98.9 Fahrenheit.

5. During a home visit, the patient tells the nurse that she feels pain in her chest when walking around the neighborhood. The nurse asks how many times it happens. The patient said just this morning. What should the nurse do?

a. Instruct the patient to sit down when experiencing this.

b. Help the patient to bed.

c. Obtain the patient's ECG.

d. Immediately administer nitroglycerin sublingually.

6. As part of the initial care and assessment of the newborn, the nurse should keep the temperature regulated by:

a. Keeping the baby in an environment with a temperature of 98.6 Fahrenheit.

b. Keeping the baby dry and wrapped in blankets.

c. Maximize the temperature of the warmer.

d. Carry and hug the baby often during the shift.

7. The nurse cleaning the newly delivered baby boy knows that she must provide airway by:

a. Suctioning nose then mouth

b. Suctioning the mouth, then nose

c. Wiping the nose and the mouth

d. Tapping the soles

8. A pregnant patient was rushed to the emergency room department with complaints of tearing sensation in her abdomen, abdominal and lower back pain, dizziness and cold clammy hands. The nurse knows that these are signs of Abruptio placenta. The nurse also knows that the patient is at risk of:

a. Idiopathic thrombocytopenic purpura

b. Thrombocytopenia

c. Deep vein thrombosis

d. Disseminated intravascular coagulation

9. In a specialty clinic, a previous patient, but newly diagnosed with HIV is asking the nurse what does Ziduvine do? The best response of the nurse is:

a. "You should probably ask the doctor as I am not allowed to discuss to you anything."

b. "It increases your immunity and resistance to the disease."

c. "It interferes with the replication of the virus."

d. "The drug usually attacks the viral wall, killing the bacteria."

10. In the ward, a patient with pneumonia asks the nurse what he can do to relieve the pain in his chest when he is coughing. The nurse advised him to:

a. Hold his cough, try deep breathing.

b. Lie flat in bed when coughing.

c. Encourage patient to decrease fluid intake.

d. Tightly hug a pillow to your chest when coughing.

11. A teenager was rushed to the hospital because of asthma attack. Upon assessment the patient has rapid, shallow breathing; 40breaths/min; some grunting sound; and flaring of the nostrils. The nurse immediately gives the patient:

   a. A glass of water to drink

   b. A bronchodilator by nebulizer

   c. Oxygen via nasal cannula

   d. Back tapping and encourage DBE.

12. The nurse knows how important APGAR score is and should assess it during:

   a. 1 to 10 minutes after delivery.

   b. 5 to 10 minutes after delivery.

   c. 1 to 5 minutes after delivery.

   d. 0 to 1 minute after delivery.

13. Nurse Leo is attending to a patient in the emergency room department, the patient suffered smoke inhalation due to a fire accident. The patient is now due for admission. After 48 hours, the patient progresses to severe hypoxia, and therefore intubated and hooked to mechanical ventilation. What could be the main condition happening to the patient?

   a. Atelectasis

   b. Pneumonia

   c. Chronic obstructive pulmonary disease

   d. Acute respiratory distress syndrome

14. The nurse is caring for a patient with chest tube. Upon inspecting the drainage, the nurse knows that the patient no longer needs it due to:

   a. Increase drainage in the tube

   b. The ABG results are all normal

   c. The patient is able to sit and stand, and with normal RR

   d. There is no longer fluctuation in the water seal chamber when suction is applied.

15. A patient that suffered from subdural hematoma is ready for discharge. Which of the following should the nurse include in her discharge plan to address the possible developing foot drop and/or contractures?

    a. Encourage the use of high-top sneakers

    b. Instruct the patient to decrease heparin intake

    c. Encourage patient to consult a physical therapist

    d. Instruct the use of the sequential compressive device

16. A patient who suffered from head trauma is expected to have increased intracranial pressure. Which of the following is the first sign to be noted?

    a. Widened pulse pressure

    b. Bradycardia

    c. Restlessness and confusion

    d. Decreased urine output

17. One of the most important protocols in every hospital after patient's delivery in identification and safety is to:

    a. Record baby's footprints in the chart.

    b. Only authorized personnel should take the newborn from the mother.

    c. Place identification bands on baby and mother.

    d. Take the APGAR score of the baby.

18. In administering phenytoin IV to the patient, the nurse knows that it should only be mixed with:

    a. Dextrose

    b. Saline solution

    c. Lactated Ringers

    d. D5 Water

19. Following the surgical repair of the patient's hip, the nurse knows that the best position to protect the leg and hip is:

    a. Pronation

    b. Supination

    c. Abduction

    d. Adduction

20. In hypothyroidism treatment, the nurse knows that this could result to which serious complication?

    a. Bone deformity

    b. Cardiac arrhythmia

    c. Thrombocytopenia

    d. Acute hemolytic reaction

21. Nurse Jek is taking care of a patient with Diabetes Insipidus. Which of the following should he prioritize as part of the treatment of the patient?

    a. Decrease fluid intake and vasopressin

    b. Increase fluid intake and vasopressin

    c. Adequate fluid intake and vasopressin

    d. Restrict fluid intake and vasopressin

22. Claris is a type I Diabetes Mellitus patient; two days ago, she acquired pneumonia and is now on hospitalization. What change will it require her?

    a. Intake of oral diabetic agents

    b. Decrease in insulin

    c. Increase in insulin

    d. No changes

23. Ruby is a 33 year old post vaginal hysterectomy. During her follow-up visit, her blood count reveals a decreased level of hematocrit. What does this mean?

    a. Infection

    b. Hemoptysis

    c. Hypovolemia

    d. Hematoma

24. In the emergency department, a patient was rushed due to partial-thickness burns to the legs and lower trunk. The nurse should anticipate which intravenous fluid?

    a. PRBC

    b. Albumin

    c. Lactated Ringer's solution

    d. D5W

25. A 55-year old male patient with congestive heart failure receives furosemide as part of his treatment. The nurse knows that this will promote, EXCEPT:

    a. An increased on the patient's urine output

    b. A decreased in pedal edema

    c. A lessened pain sensation

    d. Decreased in systolic BP

26. An important point in assessing pediatric clients is their fontanels. Which of the following statements is true regarding fontanels?

    a. Anterior fontanel is triangular shaped.

    b. Posterior fontanel is triangular shaped.

    c. Anterior fontanel closes at 6 months.

    d. Posterior fontanel closes at 1 year.

27. The nurse is giving a lecture regarding coronary artery disease. The nurse discussed about the modifiable risk factors. Which of these is the modifiable risk factor?

    a. Genes or heredity

    b. Age and gender

    c. Culture and race

    d. Weight and vices

28. The 45-year old patient was rushed to the hospital due to chest pain and DOB, further work up reveals acute myocardial infarction. Which of the following orders should the nurse question, if the patient has a history of cerebral hemorrhage?

    a. Nitroglycerin

    b. Tissue plasminogen activator

    c. Metoprolol

    d. Morphine sulfate

29. A nurse knows that a patient suffering from cardiogenic shock has the following symptoms, EXCEPT:

    a. Confusion

    b. Hypotension

    c. Tachycardia

    d. Bounding pulse

30. Taking care of the umbilical cord of the pediatric patient entails good techniques, clamping and cleaning it. The nurse knows that upon the assessment, the cord should have:

    a. Two veins and one artery

    b. Two veins and two arteries

    c. One vein and two arteries

    d. One vein and one artery

31. Nurse Len, the charge nurse in the medical ward is observing a newly assigned nurse, Pete. She asks him about what is the importance of checking the blood pressure of a patient with a history of congestive heart failure and is dyspneic. Nurse Pete should answer:

    a. It is a routine assessment of nurses.

    b. To check if progression of dyspnea.

    c. To assess pulmonary edema.

    d. To monitor heart function.

32. A clinic nurse is instructing a patient with orders of nitroglycerin to take it while sitting, and prevent standing up for at least 30 minutes. This intervention is because of the following side effects, EXCEPT:

    a. Nitroglycerin can cause hypotension.

    b. It causes headaches.

    c. It causes difficulty in breathing.

    d. It causes dizziness.

33. Cross-matching and preparation of blood units for a patient that undergoes chemotherapy is important because:

    a. There is bleeding during chemotherapy.

    b. Anemia can result from chemotherapy.

    c. Chemotherapy can cause dehydration.

    d. She needs fluid support.

34. Vicky, a vegetarian, is concerned that she is not getting enough iron from the food she eats. Knowing her condition, the nurse instructed the patient to:

    a. Instruct her to drink over the counter iron supplements.

    b. Encourage her to eat meat when her vegan friends are not looking.

    c. Advise her to use iron cookware in preparing her food.

    d. Encourage her to drink a cup of coffee or tea every meal.

ALEX RYAN & MARIE KAYE

35. A nurse is administering a blood transfusion to a patient for her treatment of anemia. The nurse knows that:

    a. Transfusion reaction happens immediately after the transfusion.

    b. Blood transfusion uses a 22G needle or IV catheter.

    c. Blood transfusion should be flushed with a dextrose solution.

    d. The nurse should remain in the room in the 15 minutes.

36. In the newborn unit, the nursing student is in charge of giving the routine newborn medications. The student nurse asks the staff nurse why the eye ointment is different from the use of another hospital. The staff nurse knows that:

    a. Their medication is the standard and should be the one followed.

    b. Other hospitals are not following the protocols.

    c. It depends on hospital policies.

    d. The ointment is the nurse's personal choice.

37. The physician has a new order of injection of Epoetin for a cancer patient. The nurse knows that Epoetin is used to:

    a. Increase the neutrophil level

    b. Increase the hematocrit level

    c. Increase the WBC count

    d. Increase iron in the blood

38. The nurse is teaching the mother of a patient with polycythemia vera. The nurse should focus on the following symptoms, EXCEPT:

    a. Decrease in the weight of the patient

    b. Increased in the clotting time

    c. Increased BP or hypertension

    d. High occurrences of headache

39. A patient is concerned about taking in corticosteroids as part of his treatment. During the interview, the nurse found out the patient has friends who took corticosteroid. The patient's concern is related to the side effect of the medications, such as, EXCEPT:

   a. Hypertension

   b. Cushingoid features

   c. Hyponatremia

   d. Low serum albumin

40. The first dose of Vitamin K is given to the newborn after delivery. The nurse knows that it is injected in the vastus lateralis and is for:

   a. To increase platelet and clotting factors.

   b. To prevent hemorrhage.

   c. To prevent infection.

   d. To increase blood count.

41. In the induction phase of chemotherapy, which of the following should the nurse focus on teaching the family members of the patient:

   a. Nutritional status of the patient.

   b. Infection control.

   c. Rest and comfort.

   d. Activities of daily living and ambulation.

42. A 5-year old, pediatric patient was admitted to the hospital due to leukemia. The nurse knows that the patient is suffering from what kind of leukemia?

   a. Acute Lymphoblastic Leukemia

   b. Chronic Lymphocytic Leukemia

   c. Acute Myelogenous Leukemia

   d. Chronic Myelogenous Leukemia

43. During the assessment, the patient in the clinic revealed to the nurse the symptoms he felt before the consultation. The nurse knows that these symptoms are typical of Hodgkin's disease. Which of the following is not a symptom of the disease?

    a. Night sweats and body weakness

    b. Fatigue and tachycardia

    c. Enlarged lymph nodes without pain

    d. Weight gain and nausea

44. The nurse is taking care of a postpartum patient. Upon checking her vital sign, the nurse noted a temperature of 100.4 Fahrenheit. The nurse knows that such reading indicates:

    a. An ongoing infection if taken in the first 24 hours postpartum.

    b. A normal reading if taken in the first 24 hours postpartum.

    c. Hemorrhage if taken in the first 24 hours postpartum.

    d. That the patient feels cold due to the delivery.

45. The nurse needs to assess the capillary refill of a sickle cell anemia patient every 2 hours. This is because:

    a. It's part of hospital policy.

    b. To check sensations of the extremities.

    c. To check any change in circulation.

    d. To assess oxygenation of extremities.

46. A patient suffering from sickle cell crisis was rushed to the hospital. The patient will be placed on the stretcher, and will be positioned:

    a. Supine

    b. Knee-chest

    c. Side lying with knees flexed

    d. Semi-fowlers with legs extended

47. One of the main goals with the patient in #46 is to prevent the progression of sickling blood cells. This could be achieved by:

   a. Administering pain relievers as ordered.

   b. Encouraging rest and sleep.

   c. Encouraging an increase of fluid intake.

   d. Preventing patient to perform ADLs.

48. A postpartum patient with her follow up check-up is concerned about her breast swelling, skin redness, tenderness in the area and is warm to touch. The nurse knows that these are signs and symptoms of Mastitis. What should the nurse instruct her to do?

   a. Encourage to rest and continue breastfeeding.

   b. Encourage to rest, but stop breastfeeding.

   c. Instruct patient to drink antibiotics and stop breastfeeding.

   d. Use only the breast not without mastitis.

49. The nurse in charge wants to check the readiness of her staff by some questions. It's nurse Lario's turn to be asked. The nurse in charge asked him, "What should be assessed in a patient with vitamin B12 deficiency?" Nurse Lario's response would be:

   a. "I should take the patient's blood pressure."

   b. "I should inspect for bleeding gums."

   c. "I should check the patient's tongue."

   d. "I should check blood results."

50. An African American patient in the E.R. has a history of bleeding. Blood count reveals that she is anemic. The sign that matches this finding is pallor. Where can the nurse check for pallor?

   a. Soles of the feet.

   b. Palm of the hands.

   c. Hard palate

   d. Conjunctiva

51. During a home visit to a 65 year old patient, the nurse noted a redness of the skin on the left side of the body. The patient told the nurse that he often sleeps on his left side. The nurse knows that this is because of:

    a. Decreased vascularity

    b. Decreased position changes

    c. Decreased skin thickness

    d. Loss of subcutaneous tissue

52. A patient with idiopathic thrombocytpenic purpura undergoing treatment is wondering why there is a need to get some blood sample. The best response by the nurse would be:

    a. "To check your platelet count."

    b. "To check your WBC count."

    c. "To check your clotting time."

    d. "To check your RBS count."

53. During a follow-up check-up of a patient with autoimmune thrombocytopenic purpura, the physician orders for a CBC test. The result shows a platelet count of 10,000. The patient is due for admission. The nurse should instruct the patient and family relatives about:

    a. Risk of injury due to dizziness.

    b. Risk of infection.

    c. Risk of bleeding.

    d. Risk of loss of consciousness.

54. The nurse is receiving a post-transsphenoidal hypophysectomy patient. The nurse should anticipate that the position of the patient would be:

    a. Trendelenburg

    b. Knee-chest position

    c. Semi-fowler's position

    d. Pronation

55. During a home visit to a 58-year old patient, the nurse saw signs of decreased skin vascularity. Which of the following is the effect of this finding?

    a. Increased diastolic blood pressure.

    b. Altered thermoregulation.

    c. Altered skin turgor.

    d. Increased perception of pain.

56. Nurse Dan is doing his nursing rounds when a patient cried for help due to epistaxis. Which of the following would help control the bleeding?

    a. Instruct the patient sit straight, hyperextend his neck and pinch the soft area of the nose.

    b. Get gauze pads and pack it in the patient's nostrils.

    c. Place the patient in a sitting position, head bowed down while pinching the soft area of the nose.

    d. Place ice packs, one on the forehead, and one on the nape.

57. The nurse should monitor the blood pressure of a patient that has undergone a tumor removal by unilateral adrenalectomy. This is because:

    a. An indicator of infection.

    b. An indicator of cardiac output.

    c. An indicator of cardiovascular collapse.

    d. An indicator of urine output.

58. Mr. Sam is admitted due to tremor and pallor. He had been vomiting for the past 3 days prior to hospitalization and has difficulty eating. He was given IV glucocorticoids. An important intervention for the patient is:

    a. Continuous glucometer reading as ordered.

    b. Strict Input and Output measurement and recordings.

    c. Routine blood tests, especially hematocrit level.

    d. Assessment of skin for edema and turgor.

59. In the surgical ward the nurse assesses a patient first day post total thyroidectomy. The patient complains of pins and needle feeling around her mouth and fingers. The nurse knows that this is an effect of:

 a. Decreased serum calcium

 b. Decreased serum glucose

 c. Decreased serum potassium

 d. Decreased thyroid hormone

60. A 36-year old patient is diagnosed of hypothyroidism. The nurse knows that the causes of this condition are, EXCEPT:

 a. Hashimoto's thyroiditis

 b. Thyroidectomy

 c. Radioactive Iodine treatment

 d. Grave's disease

61. A 28-year old female suffering from migraine told the nurse that she drinks several medications (2 kinds of analgesics) to relieve the pain she is feeling. The nurse knows that the patient is at risk of:

 a. Overdose

 b. Polypharmacy

 c. Blood Dyscrasia

 d. Autoimmune diseases

62. In question #61 what percentage is the patient at risk of having adverse effects of the medication she is taking?

 a. 6%

 b. 36%

 c. 100%

 d. 65%

63. The nurse is accompanying a patient for an arteriogram. The patient told the nurse that he is feeling hot. The nurse responds by saying:

    a. "I will tell the physician to stop the procedure right away."

    b. "Don't worry; I will give you some Benadryl."

    c. "There is no need to worry, as that feeling is normal."

    d. "The warmth you are feeling means that you are getting better."

64. The head nurse in her staff on the different ward procedures to test their knowledge. Which of the following actions needs further teaching?

    a. The LPN donned gloves before giving a patient a bath.

    b. The RN wears protective eye gear before getting a blood sample from the patient.

    c. The physician washes his hands before and after examining the patient.

    d. The staff nurse donned gloves before taking vital signs.

65. A patient diagnosed to have bipolar is undergoing electorconvulsive therapy (ECT). To assess for the effectiveness of the treatment, the patient should:

    a. Fall asleep

    b. Have a headache

    c. Have increased HR and BP

    d. Have a grand mal seizure

66. A mother is concerned that her 3-year son might have worms inside him. She told the clinic nurse that she always sees her child scratching his anus. The nurse instructed the mother to:

    a. Send a stool sample to the lab.

    b. Check the anus of her child 2-3 hours after he sleeps using a flashlight.

    c. Scrape the area with a tongue depressor

    d. Prescribe a medication for the worm infection.

67. In the community discussion, the nurse is lecturing the community folks regarding Enterobiasis. Which of the following responses will indicate that the community folks understood Enterobiasis?

a. "Children less than 10 years of age are prone to these worms."

b. "The whole household should be treated."

c. "The child needs to be compliant for the 1 year treatment."

d. "Noncompliance with medication will result to admission."

68. A post total thyroidectomy patient on her follow-up check-up asked the nurse on food sources of vitamin D. The nurse should respond with:

a. Cereals, clams, and dried fruit

b. Apricots, bananas, and broccoli

c. Creamed soups, clams and spinach

d. Egg-yolk, milk, and ketchup

69. The charge nurse in a cancer ward is making assignments for her staff. One of the nurses is pregnant, what patient condition should she assign to her?

a. A patient with a treatment of linear acceleration radiation therapy.

b. A patient with radium implant

c. A patient who has soluble brachytherapy

d. A patient who has iridium seeds

70. In the medical ward, the ER has phoned in 4 admissions for a private room. There is only one vacant room available in the ward. Which case should the nurse place in the private room?

a. A patient diagnosed with Cushing's disease

b. A patient with type II Diabetes Mellitus

c. A patient with acromegaly

d. A patient with hyperthyroidism

71. The nurse is the neonatal intensive care unit administered an adult dose of IV digoxin to a newborn. The nurse without checking the dosage administered the medication and as a result the newborn suffers a permanent brain and heart damage. The nurse now faces what offense?

    a. Negligence

    b. Malpractice

    c. Assault

    d. Tort

72. A newly assigned LPN is performing some ward routines. Which of the following should she do?

    a. Inserting a Foley catheter.

    b. Start a blood transfusion.

    c. Administering IV medications.

    d. Starting nebulization of the patient.

73. In the recovery room of the operating room, the nurse doing the assessment of vital signs got the following: BP-90/50 mmHg, PR-134 bpm, RR-32. What should the nurse's first priority?

    a. Monitor the vital signs every 30 minutes.

    b. Notify the physician and anticipate new orders.

    c. Assess patient's level of consciousness.

    d. Increase the IV infusion rate.

74. A newly admitted patient diagnosed with diverticulosis asked the nurse what food should be avoided. The nurse response is:

    a. Avoid fatty foods.

    b. Avoid caffeine, chocolates, and mints.

    c. Avoid low-residue diet.

    d. Limit sodium intake.

75. Which of the following nurses is more knowledgeable in taking care of a patient with pre-eclampsia?

    a. With 6 weeks experience in the postpartum unit.

    b. With 2 years experience in the maternal care unit.

    c. With 5 years' experience in the surgical area.

    d. With a Master's degree in maternal and child care, fresh graduate.

76. Nurse Cath asked her patient if he took his medications. The client answered her, "Yes." In the recording of medications, Nurse Cath signed the medications, even if she is not the one who administers the medications. The charge nurse seeing this should:

    a. Talk to the nurse and call the Board of Nursing

    b. Issue a written reprimand and terminate the nurse

    c. Talk to the nurse and file a formal reprimand

    d. Report the incident as a case of Tort

77. A group of community health nurses is planning on their Monday home visits. Which of the following patients should they visit last?

    a. A patient with MRSA with Vancomycin treatment via PICC line

    b. A patient with an exacerbation of multiple sclerosis

    c. A pediatric patient with pneumonia

    d. An elderly patient with PEG tube due to gastrectomy

78. A patient newly diagnosed with Alzheimer's disease in a homecare unit has the following symptoms: profound memory deficits, inability to concentrate or manage activities of daily living. The nurse knows that this stage is:

    a. Stage I

    b. Stage II

    c. Stage III

    d. Stage IV

79. The nurse is caring for an 8-year old child with a diagnosis of conjunctivitis, now on his 2nd day of hospitalization. What intervention should be done before administering eye drops?

   a. Clean the patient's eye with warm water.

   b. Allow the parents to instill the medication.

   c. Instruct the patient on how to instill the medication.

   d. Assess for redness and edema, if not present do not give the medication.

80. A 1 and a half year old child was brought to the hospital due to on and off fever and vomiting. The physician will be examining the child further. Which of the following should the nurse do?

   a. Instruct the parents to leave the room.

   b. Talk with the parents in order for them to lose focus and not look at their child during assessment.

   c. Encourage the patient to stay with the child.

   d. Get the crying child away from his parents in order to start the assessment.

81. The nurse is giving an instruction on how to maintain hearing-aid. Which of the following is NOT correct?

   a. Clean the hearing-aid every day.

   b. Store the hearing-aid in a cool, dry place.

   c. Clean the hearing aid with a soft material.

   d. Check the batteries if functioning properly.

82. Nurse Eva is caring for a 13-year old patient post-tonsillectomy. Which of the following should she prioritize?

   a. Altered nutrition

   b. Body image disturbance

   c. Risk for aspiration

   d. Pain

83. The nurse is preparing a discharge instruction for a patient with Asthma. Which of the following should NOT be included in the instructions?

　　a. Provide an instruction on the proper use of metered-dose inhalers.

　　b. Instruct the patient and the family about the triggering agents.

　　c. Instruct the patient to limit fluids to 2L/day

　　d. Instruct patient to seek immediate medical attention if symptoms are not relieved by medications.

84. A pediatric patient was rushed to the hospital due to fever and productive cough. The nurse considers these as signs of what disease?

　　a. Bacterial pneumonia

　　b. Viral pneumonia

　　c. Rhinitis

　　d. Asthma

85. A 6-year old patient is admitted due to epiglottitis. The nurse should anticipate the need and the risks involved and prepared this at the bedside:

　　a. Sedation set

　　b. Tracheostomy set

　　c. Oxygen paraphernalia

　　d. Intravenous access supplies

86. A patient went to the consulting unit, upon the interview; the nurse noted any observable signs from the patient and recognized these as Grave's disease. Which of the following is not a symptom of the condition?

　　a. Exophthalmia

　　b. Fine, straight hair

　　c. Thin body built

　　d. Pale skin

87. A mother is concerned on the nutritional intake of her child with celiac disease. The nurse understanding the need for instruction tells the mother of the food her child can take. The mother shows her understanding by responding:

    a. "I should always prepare sandwich as his snack in school."

    b. "I should prepare pasta, even just once a day."

    c. "He can have pancakes and doughnuts once a week."

    d. "I should prepare omelets and milk products.

88. The nurse is conducting a lecture to teenagers and women regarding breast self-examination. The recipients of the lecture show understanding by:

    a. "I should do BSE with the help of others."

    b. "I should palpate first before observing."

    c. "I have to perform BSE once a month."

    d. "I have to do BSE during my monthly period."

89. A gravida 4 para 1 patient is admitted to the maternity unit and will undergo amniotomy. The nurse should expect:

    a. A moderate amount of reddish fluid.

    b. A small amount of greenish fluid.

    c. A moderate amount of straw-colored fluid.

    d. A small amount of white fluid.

90. The Testicular Cancer Research Center recommends that males should also perform a monthly TSE. Which of the following is the correct information about this?

    a. The testicles should have the same approximate size, if one is larger, seek medical help.

    b. Self-examination is best performed after a warm bath or shower.

    c. Examine each testicle with both hands.

    d. Lumps on the epididymis are not cancerous.

91. The nurse is monitoring a pregnant patient in the labor room. During assessment she has the following: 8cm dilation, FHR of 170, variability of 0-2bpm. The nurse indicates that these are signs of what type of deceleration?

    a. Early deceleration

    b. Late deceleration

    c. Variable deceleration

    d. No deceleration

92. In checking the fetal heart rate, the nurse knows that there are factors affecting it. Which of the following statement defines a normal fetal heart rate?

    a. The normal range is 170-190bpm with an average of 180bpm.

    b. The normal baseline variability is 35-45 in the monitor.

    c. Ominous changes are present.

    d. FHR increases with fetal movements.

93. A 57-year old male was rushed to the hospital due to difficulty of breathing and a bluish color of the lips. Work-ups are done which revealed left-sided heart failure. Which of the following are signs of Left-sided heart failure?
    I. Orthopnea
    II. Tachycardia
    III. JVD
    IV. Wheezes

    a. I, II, III

    b. I, III, IV

    c. II, III, IV

    d. II, IV, I

94. The nurse in the family planning clinic is discussing about the methods of family planning to a couple. Which response made by the clients' shows understanding of the rhythm method?

a. "It is effective only below 35 years of age for women and 40 years for men."

b. "It is effective in counting the intercourse in a month."

c. "It depends on the regularity of the menstrual cycle."

d. "We should check her temperature before having intercourse."

95. A diabetic woman went to the family planning clinic for a consultation. She wanted to know the best family planning method for her case. The family planning nurse recommends:

a. Oral contraceptives

b. Contraceptive sponge

c. IUD

d. Diaphragm

96. A pregnant woman on her 20th week of pregnancy was rushed to the hospital. The physician suspects a case of ectopic pregnancy. Which of the following signs supports the diagnosis of the physician?

a. Painful vaginal bleeding

b. Painless vaginal bleeding

c. Abdominal contractions and pain

d. Sharp, lower abdominal pain

97. On her monthly check-up a pregnant woman in her second trimester of pregnancy is concerned that she still vomits and feels nauseated most of the time. She was admitted due to hyperemesis gravidarum. The nurse knows that the patient is at risk of developing:

a. Metabolic alkalosis with dehydration.

b. Metabolic acidosis with dehydration.

c. Respiratory alkalosis without dehydration.

d. Respiratory acidosis without dehydration.

98. Some women are thought to be pregnant because of a big belly. While others are really pregnant, but it does not show, such in the case of Stef. She is a primigravida and is 20 weeks pregnant. What is the best proof of her pregnancy?

    a. Uterine enlargement

    b. Increase in breast size

    c. Presence of fetal heart tones

    d. Presence of movement in the abdomen

99. A student nurse was given the assignment of taking care of a COPD patient. The nurse supervising the student asks her to teach the patient on ways to decrease air trapping. Which of these actions should the student nurse teach?

    a. Deep breathing exercises

    b. Coughing exercises

    c. Pursed-lip breathing

    d. Rhythmic breathing

100. 24 hours after the delivery of a baby boy, the doctor prescribed RhoGam injection to the mother. It shows that the mother is Rh negative and the baby is positive. When is the most efficient time to administer the injection?

    a. Within 72 hours after delivery

    b. Within a week

    c. Within 2 weeks

    d. Within 3 weeks

ANSWERS:

1. Correct Answer: C.

Breastfeeding does not relieve the pain in childbirth, as the pain may be caused by the cut in the perineum made during delivery. This is relieved by pain medications. However, breastfeeding makes the choices A, B and D.

2. Correct Answer: C.

This is a kind of fungus that is transmitted to humans by birds. By interview, you may be able to find out if the patient has been exposed to birds, or caring some birds.

3. Correct Answer: B.

An abdominal aortic aneurysm that is increasing in size and is at risk of rupture causes lower back pain. Choice A is mostly related to cardio disease. Choice C and D are neurologic.

4. Correct Answer: A.

Cardiac Output is a result of stroke volume x Heart Rate. If the BP of the patient is within the normal range, then that is the best indicator, as sufficient cardiac output results in blood pressure within normal range. Choice C and D are not related to the heart.

5. Correct Answer: A.

The patient should immediately stop walking and sit, this is to minimize oxygen consumption and work of the heart. If pain persists, then nitroglycerin should be given then the ECG (if portable ones are available with the nurse). Do not assist her to go back to bed, as walking will again cause the pain.

6. Correct Answer: B.

The baby should be kept warm with the use of clothes, warmer in regulated temperature and blankets. Choice A is not necessary. Choice C will result in a toasted baby. Choice D, although tempting, will not keep the baby warm at all times.

7. Correct Answer: C.

In accordance with the latest research that suctioning causes bradycardia, it is no longer advised. Wiping the nose and the mouth, followed by a gentle stimulation of the patient's back will help provide airway.

8. Correct Answer: D.

Abruptio placenta can cause hemorrhage and can be concealed, therefore the patient can develop DIC due to the activation of the clotting cascade. Choice A has no definitive cause. Choice B is a decreased in platelet number. And choice C is caused by stagnation of blood in the veins causing thrombus formation.

9. Correct Answer: C.

Ziduvine is prescribed to newly diagnosed HIV patient to prevent the virus from becoming numerous by hindering the replication process. It does not destroy the viral cell wall, nor does it increase the patient's immunity. Choice A is definitely wrong as the nurse is capable of explaining it to the patient.

10. Correct Answer: D.

Hugging a pillow to the chest is a splitting technique that helps the diaphragm when coughing. Therefore, it will relieve the pain felt. Choice A will not be effective as a cough is a reflex. Choice B will make it difficult to breath and will promote coughing. Choice C is wrong as fluids are encouraged.

11. Correct Answer: B.

The patient is already exhibiting respiratory distress; therefore a bronchodilator should be given immediately. This will open the airways and maximize the oxygen inhalation. Other choices will not alleviate the problem.

12. Correct Answer: C.

It is important to get the APGAR score in the most vital minutes of life and that is 1-5 minutes after delivery. If you wait until 10 minutes, environmental factors will already affect the baby, such as the baby's first bath.

13. Correct Answer: D.

Fire and smoke inhalation causes severe hypoxia, which is a typical sign of ARDS. Choice A, B, and C are not related to fire and smoke.

14. Correct Answer: D.

A chest tube is to help in the re-expansion of the lung and maintain that expansion. If no longer fluctuating it means that the lung has expanded and remained expanded. Further test, such as X-ray should reveal the same.

15. Correct Answer: A.

This is the best solution to prevent foot drop and contractures and the only choice in the given that is specifically made for foot.

16. Correct Answer: C.

The first sign seen in the patient is always the level of consciousness. Widened pulse pressure, bradycardia and decreased urine output can develop later.

17. Correct Answer: C.

For identification and infant safety, identification bands should be placed on the baby and mother immediately after delivery.

18. Correct Answer: B.

The safest that will not interact or cause damage to the medication, phenytoin, is saline solution. The other fluids can interact with the medicine such as the dextrose that can cause the medicine to crystallize.

19. Correct Answer: C.

The hips and legs are placed near to each other, this is an abduction. It helps in the stabilization of prosthesis placed in the acetabulum.

20. Correct Answer: B.

The electrolyte involves is calcium and is part of the contraction of the heart. Therefore, the nurse should monitor for signs of cardiac arrhythmias.

21. Correct Answer: C.

The main goal in the treatment is to provide adequate fluid intake (to maintain normal function of the body, do not decrease, increase or restrict) and vasopressin.

22. Correct Answer: C.

A Diabetic patient that has acquired an infection needs to increase her insulin intake due to the stress on her body. This is called compensation due to the increased level of blood glucose.

23. Correct Answer: D.

This a delayed complication of the procedure which presents as a decreased hematocrit level.

24. Correct Answer: C.

The patient needs fluid as well as electrolyte support that could be given by the LRS. The most important electrolyte support is to replenish sodium. It will also correct metabolic acidosis in the patient.

25. Correct Answer: C.

Furosemide is given to patients who need to decrease fluid in the body. Therefore, the results are choices A, B, and D. Furosemide is not related to managing pain.

26. Correct Answer: B.

Here are your fontanel facts: Anterior fontanel is diamond-shaped and closes at 12 to 18 months. The posterior fontanel is triangular in and closes at 2 to 3 months.

27. Correct Answer: D.

Weight and vices are part of lifestyle, and therefore can be controlled and changed. Choices A, B, and C are not modifiable risk factors.

28. Correct Answer: B.

Tissue plasminogen activator (tPA) prevents aggregation of platelets and dissolves clots by converting plasminogen to plasmin.

29. Correct Answer: D.

Cardiogenic shock results from overworked heart to keep the equilibrium in the body. Therefore the heart no longer functions well and results to decrease in blood flow to the different organs, especially the brain. The signs are confusion, hypotension, tachycardia and weak pulse.

30. Correct Answer: C.

A pediatric umbilical cord contains one vein and two arteries. The vein carries oxygenated blood, while the arteries carry unoxygenated blood.

31. Correct Answer: C.

A patient with a history of congestive heart failure who is now dyspneic may already have pulmonary edema. As a result the patient will have severe hypertension.

32. Correct Answer: C.

Nitroglycerin is a potent vasodilator which has the following side effects: hypotension, headaches, dizziness, but not difficulty in breathing.

33. Correct Answer: B.

Chemotherapy suppresses bone-marrow, our blood-producing organ. Therefore, it can cause anemia. Blood transfusion of compatible blood is needed after a complete blood count has been done.

34. Correct Answer: C.

Iron cookware are proven efficient in adding iron to food, especially to the vegetables being cooked using it. You cannot force the patient to eat or drink something that is against her beliefs.

35. Correct Answer: D.

Transfusion reaction has a greater chance of happening in the first 15 minutes of the blood transfusion. Therefore the nurse should keep a keen eye and monitor the vital signs of the patient to ensure that transfusion reaction will be prevented.

36. Correct Answer: C.

The antibiotic ointment used in the eye of the newborn depends on the hospital policies and does not depend on choices A, B, and D.

37. Correct Answer: B.

Epoetin is actually an erythropoietin, which is necessary for the production of RBCs. The result is an increased level of hematocrit.

38. Correct Answer: A.

Polycythemia vera means that there is an overproduction of RBCs by the bone marrow. Therefore, there is an increased hematocrit and viscosity of the blood. Therefore, it does not affect the weight of the patient.

39. Correct Answer: C.

Corticosteroid therapy has the following common side effects fluid retention (resulting in weight gain, hypertension and fluid retention), cushingoid features (or moonface feature), and low serum albumin.

40. Correct Answer: B.

Vitamin K is given to prevent hemorrhage in newborn clients as they are cut away from their uterine protection.

41. Correct Answer: B.

In the induction phase of chemotherapy, the patient is highly immunocompromised. The nurse should focus on infection control, not just for the patient, but for the visitors as well. This includes not bringing fresh fruits, vegetables, and other fresh things because they might carry microbes. Hand washing and the wearing of protective gears should also be implemented.

42. Correct Answer: A.

ALL is the most common leukemia in ages 3 years up to 10 years old. Choice B and C affect 60 years old and above. Choice D affects ages 45 to 55 years old.

43. Correct Answer: D.

The usual symptoms of Hodgkin's disease are: night sweats, body malaise/weakness, fatigue, tachycardia, enlarged cervical lymph nodes without pain, and weight loss. Therefore choice D are not symptoms.

44. Correct Answer: B.

A slight increase in the temperature within the first 24 hours postpartum is normal (100.4 Fahrenheit). If the temperature is greater than 101.4 Fahrenheit, then that should be considered as an infection.

45. Correct Answer: C.

In sickle cell anemia, there could be an occlusion of the blood vessels, therefore a change in his capillary refill (should be less than 3 seconds) would indicate a change in circulation. Sickle cell anemia may have a good SPO2 reading, therefore choice D is wrong. Choices A and B is not related to the disease.

46. Correct Answer: D.

In sickle cell crisis, the main priority is to provide oxygenation. The best position therefore is a relaxed body that allows the circulation of blood better. And this can be seen in semi-fowler's position (more lung expansion for better oxygenation) with legs extended on bed for better circulation.

47. Correct Answer: C.

Increasing the hydration of the patient will decrease the sickling of the blood cells. The recommended fluid intake of the patient should be 200ml every hour and could come in any form –water, juice, popsicle, and others.

48. Correct Answer: A.

Mastitis is an inflammation of the mammary glands and can occur in the first several weeks of breastfeeding, or anytime during breastfeeding. Antibiotics are prescribed and should be taken by the patient. The breast milk is not infected and will not harm the infant.

49. Correct Answer: C.

A patient who has vit. B12 deficiency has a smooth and beefy red tongue. Therefore, choice A, B, and D are incorrect.

50. Correct Answer: C.

Hard palate is the best part of the body to be checked as it does not differ in color with the other races. You would expect a darker color of the skin of the African American, and at times yellow palms, soles and conjunctiva.

51. Correct Answer: C.

Elderly patients are more prone to skin breakdown due to decreased skin thickness. Therefore the nurse should frequently assess for signs of pressure ulcers.

52. Correct Answer: A.

A patient with this disease has decreased platelet count. In order to assess the effectiveness of his treatment, checking of platelet count should be done.

53. Correct Answer: C.

A platelet count of less than 20,000 already make the patient prone to bleeding. The normal platelet count ranges from 120,000 to 400,000. Choice A is a probable risk factor for decreased RBC. Choice C for decreased WBC. And choice D is not related.

54. Correct Answer: C.

To relieve intracranial pressure, the best position is semi-fowler's position. Choice A, B, and D will only increase the ICP.

55. Correct Answer: B.

One of the changes in the elderly skin is decreased skin vascularity. This result to altered thermoregulation and increased risk for heat stroke.

56. Correct Answer: C.

The patient should sit upright, head bowed down to prevent the ingestion of blood. Pinch the soft area of the nose for approximately 5 minutes or more for clotting purposes. Place the ice pack directly on the nose, and the nape.

57. Correct Answer: C.

Blood pressure will tell so much of the function of adrenal gland such as the function of the cardiovascular system. This is because the remaining gland can be affected by the tumor removal; therefore, its function might be suppressed.

58. Correct Answer: A.

IV glucocorticoids have the tendency of increasing the blood glucose level, which might need additional intervention, such as insulin. The patient does not require choices B, C, and D as it will not determine the effect of the medication.

59. Correct Answer: A.

In total thyroidectomy the parathyroid gland, which is responsible for the regulation of serum calcium, might be affected. It may not function well after the surgery and may take several months to regain its normal functioning, most especially if it was relocated. The signs presented are the typical sign of decreased serum calcium.

60. Correct Answer: D.

Grave's disease is a common case of hyperthyroidism. All the other choices are causes of hypothyroidism.

61. Correct Answer: B.

Polypharmacy is defined as the concurrent use of several drugs. The number of drug use determines the rate of adverse effect felt by the patient.

62. Correct Answer: A.

The given ratio for 2 medications taken is 6%, for 8 medications is considered 100%. The two other percentages are ratios done to predict the 4 medications and 6 medications.

63. Correct Answer: C.

In arteriogram, a dye is used for the examination. The patient will normally feel warm when the dye is injected, but it does not mean the patient is having an allergic reaction.

64. Correct Answer: D.

There is no need to wear gloves before taking the vital signs of a patient. The nurse should only wear gloves if the patient has a skin infection such as methicillin-resistant staphylococcus aureus.

65. Correct Answer: D.

An effective ECT will exhibit with the patient having grand mal seizure. The seizure indicates that the neurons are shifting.

66. Correct Answer: B.

Scratching the perianal area is a sign that the child might have pinworms. The best way to assess the condition is for the parent to examine the area when the child is asleep, preferable 2-3 hours after. She must use a flashlight and use a clear tape to get samples of the eggs/worms.

67. Correct Answer: B.

To ensure that there is no infestation within the family and those interacting in the household, such as the helpers, everybody should be treated.

68. Correct Answer: C.

The food set is considered calcium-rich foods. While choice A is iron-rich, choice B is potassium-rich and choice D is low-sodium foods.

69. Correct Answer: A.

Any pregnant woman, whether a nurse or not, should not be exposed to any radiation. The safest client for the pregnant nurse is choice A as the procedure is done in the radium department and stays there. The patient will just come back to the ward when the radiation is no longer harmful to other patients.

70. Correct Answer: A.

The charge nurse should prioritize the patient that is immunocompromised when assigning rooms. This is a case wherein the adrenal cortex is not functioning well. The other choices do not show risk of infection and are not immunocompromised.

71. Correct Answer: B.

Malpractice is a result of an action disregarding knowledge that resulted to harm to the patient. Choice A is not caring for the patient, or not performing the nurse's duties. Choice C is physical and/or verbal attack. And choice D is an illegal act involving the patient's belongings.

72. Correct Answer: A.

The LPN can perform this task with or without the supervision of the nurse. However, she cannot administer medication and start blood transfusion.

73. Correct Answer: B.

The vital signs show that the condition of the patient is deteriorating, therefore it needs to be reported to the physician for interventions. Choice A is a protocol in the recovery room, but will not help the patient's situation. Choice C is not effective as the patient still has anesthesia effects. And choice D should not be done without doctor's orders.

74. Correct Answer: C.

A patient with diverticulosis is instructed to increase fiber diet in order to help clean the intestines and to prevent furthering of the disease. Choice A is for Cholelithiasis. Choice B is for Gastroesophageal reflux. And choice D is for Nephrotic syndrome.

75. Correct Answer: B.

The experience is still the best teacher and is exhibited by the RN in choice B. Although choice D has a Master's degree, she is still a fresh graduate, therefore her practical exposure is lesser, although she knows the concepts and theories behind. Choice A has less experience than choice B. And choice C is not related to maternal care.

76. Correct Answer: C.

The incident should be reported by filing a formal reprimand to the Nursing Service Department of the Hospital who will study the case of the nurse.

77. Correct Answer: A.

Among the cases, the most infectious should be seen last in order to avoid cross infection of other patients.

78. Correct Answer: B.

This is the most common stage when the disease is actually diagnosed and are characterized as the mentioned symptoms. Stage I usually has loss of short term memory and irritability. Stage II has aphasia and inability to recognize or use objects. And stage IV the patient becomes nonverbal and completely withdrawn.

79. Correct Answer: A.

The nurse is responsible in giving the medication not the child or the parents. Clean the patient's eyes first and remove any exudates. The eye drop should only be stopped as per order.

80. Correct Answer: C.

To the child, the health practitioners are strangers, and during the time of sickness the parents serve as comfort. Let the patient stay with the child. Some would even ask the assistance of the mother in carrying the child, so as not to cry while the assessment in on-going.

81. Correct Answer: B.

Hearing-aids should be stored in a warm and dry place. Choice A, C and D are correct.

82. Correct Answer: C.

In prioritizing nursing diagnoses it is important to follow tips, in this case ABC is more important than Maslow's hierarchy of needs. Risk of aspiration therefore should be prioritize first as it can hinder airway.

83. Correct Answer: C.

Asthma is a condition in the lungs; therefore, fluid intake is not part of the discharge instructions. Cases that concern fluids are mostly cardiovascular diseases.

84. Correct Answer: A.

Bacterial pneumonia exhibits as an infection that causes high fever and productive cough. Viral pneumonia shows rhinitis, headache, cough, and body weakness. Asthma has wheezing and shortness of breath.

85. Correct Answer: B.

The main concern in patients with epiglottitis is airway obstruction. The tracheostomy set is needed in case the need for airway.

86. Correct Answer: D.

Grave's disease is also known as hyperthyroidism. In which the patient experiences the following observable signs: fine, straight hair; bulging eyes (exophthalmos); facial blushing; enlarged thyroid; weight loss; muscle wasting; clubbing of fingernails; and tremors.

87. Correct Answer: D.

Patient's with Celiac disease should have gluten-free diets. Gluten is found in breads and wheat products.

88. Correct Answer: C.

Brest self-examination should be done once a month, preferably after menstruation. The woman should stand in front of a mirror and observe for symmetry, lumps and others; then palpate; then lean forward.

89. Correct Answer: C.

Amniotomy is a procedure to rupture the amniotic sac/membrane to initiate labor. The normal color of the fluid should be straw-colored. A greenish fluid might indicate meconium staining. The reddish and white fluid is just made up.

90. Correct Answer: A.

It is normal for one testicle to be larger than the other. Choices B, C, and D are correct. Cancerous lumps are usually found on the sides of the testicle.

91. Correct Answer: B.

Late decelerations are linked to uteroplacental deficiency, which is a result of uterine contractions. This means that there isn't enough oxygen reaching the child and causes fetal tachycardia,

92. Correct Answer: D.

The normal FHR is 110-160bpm. The normal variability is 5-25. Ominous means threatening. Therefore D is the correct answer.

93. Correct Answer: D.

Left-sided heart failure exhibits pulmonary signs with dysrhythmias and tachycardia. JVD is a sign of right-sided heart failure.

94. Correct Answer: C.

Rhythm method is also called the calendar method as it depends on the menstrual cycle of the woman to keep track of the ovulation and the "safe" days.

95. Correct Answer: D.

in recommending the best method, you should take in consideration the case of the patient. Oral contraceptives will increase glucose in her blood. Contraceptive sponge has less effectiveness for the patient. IUD may cause inflammation.

96. Correct Answer: D.

The common symptoms of ectopic pregnancy are light vaginal bleeding, nausea and vomiting with pain, and sharp abdominal cramps/lower abdominal pain. Choice A is abruption placenta. Choice B is placenta previa. Choice D is labor.

97. Correct Answer: B.

The patient is at risk of dehydration as she keeps on vomiting. This dehydration is the precursor in having metabolic acidosis in the patient.

98. Correct Answer: C.

At 20 weeks AOG, fetal heart tones can already be appreciated and is the best proof of pregnancy. As in the case presented a primigravida can actually have a smaller uterine size. Choice B can also happen during the menstrual cycle. And choice D can be affected by other factors.

99. Correct Answer: C.

Pursed-lip breathing is breathing out through a pursed-lip, therefore decreasing air trapping. Choice A is done to help patients who have SOB. Choice B is for the patient who has difficulty expelling phlegm. And choice D is for pregnant women in labor.

100. Correct Answer: A.

RhoGam should be administered within 72 hours after delivery because the mother was exposed to the blood cells of the baby.

III. NCLEX Exam Three

QUESTIONS:

1. A 52-year old patient was brought to the emergency room due to shortness of breath. Further assessment reveals bounding pulse, dysrhythmia based on ECG, and dependent edema. The nurse suspects a heart problem, which is:

    a. Coronary Artery Disease

    b. Right-sided Heart Failure

    c. Left-sided Heart Failure

    d. Myocardial Infarction

2. The nurse in the nursery is taking care of a newborn of an addicted mother. The nurse knows that the newborn would undergo withdrawal, a case known as a narcotic abstinence syndrome. An important nursing intervention is:

    a. To instruct the mother to carry the newborn.

b. To provide an area where the newborn will hear sounds.

c. To wrap the baby comfortably with a blanket.

d. To instruct the mother to frequently provide a tactile stimulation.

3. Many pregnant patients opt to have epidural anesthesia because of the alleviation of pain during labor and delivery. The nurse understands this option, and knows the intervention to be performed, which is:

a. Assess for the blood pressure.

b. Frequent assessment of cervical dilation.

c. Monitor fetal heart rate

d. Encourage patient to remain in a lying position.

4. Before attending to the needs of a post-operative patient, the nurse should what technique to prevent infection of the wound?

a. Use alcohol or disinfectant and rub it until it dries.

b. Perform proper hand washing.

c. Wear mask and protective eye gear.

d. Minimize contact with the patient.

5. Every Monday, the clinic nurse teaches patients while they wait for their consultation. This time the topic is Diabetes. Which of the following statements is NOT true about Diabetes Mellitus?

a. It is a chronic metabolic disorder marked by hyperglycemia.

b. It can result from a primary failure of pancreatic alpha cells to produce insulin.

c. It can result from the development of insulin resistance in body cells.

d. There are two main types of Diabetes: Type 1 and Type 2.

6. A 55-year old patient arrived in the emergency room department with complaints of hip pain and bruising in the area. The relatives revealed that the patient fell while going down the stairs (with 5 steps). The physician suspects a hip fracture. Which of the following supports that notion?

   a. Localized pain

   b. Observable misalignment.

   c. Cool extremity.

   d. Unappreciated pedal pulses.

7. The nurse is teaching in a class of women regarding osteoporosis. Mrs. Sy, 57 years of age, is listening intently to the lecture. She shows her understanding by responding:

   a. "I need to exercise more as lack of exercise is the main cause of osteoporosis."

   b. "Menopausal women are more prone to developing osteoporosis."

   c. "I need to drink calcium supplements, as I age, my serum calcium decreases."

   d. "Osteoporosis is likely to happen if my mother and grandmother before had it."

8. A Bryant's traction was used to help in the quick recovery of a pediatric patient who underwent repair of a fractured right femur. In order to know that the traction is working properly, the nurse should be able to observe:

   a. The child is able to move his left leg.

   b. The child's buttocks are 15° off from the bed.

   c. There are pins secured properly.

   d. The leg is suspended in the traction.

9. A 24-year old male is placed on a Balanced Skeletal Traction due to fracture of femur. The traction is necessary to:

   a. Align the pedal bones with the tibia.

   b. Reduce painful muscle spasms.

   c. Heal the legs immediately.

   d. Prevent hip extension contractures.

10. A cheerleader was rushed to the hospital after an accident during their practice. The doctor advised for an ORIF (open reduction internal fixation) procedure of her left hip. Immediately after the surgery, the nurse gives priority to:

    a. Engaging client to physical therapy.

    b. Assessing pain.

    c. The nutritional intake.

    d. Assessing the serum collection (Davol) drain.

11. In the emergency department, a relative watching over his patient approaches the nurse and asked if she could take his BP. The nurse agreed to take his BP, which is 140/80mmHg. The watcher said, "Oh, I have hypertension." The nurse should respond:

    a. "Definitely, I think you should go for a check-up."

    b. "When was the last time your BP was taken and what was the result?"

    c. "We have emergency medications for you."

    d. "Do you have any maintenance medication you can take right now?"

12. The nurse is teaching the wife of a patient with a percutaneous gastrostomy tube on the proper feeding techniques. Which of the following responses shows her understanding?

    a. "I should always flush the tube with drinking water after each feeding and clamp the tube after."

    b. "There is a need to check the placement of the tube three times a day, to prevent removal."

    c. "I will immediately notify the physician if I see signs of indigestion."

    d. "If he has difficulty in swallowing, I will stop the feeding and bring him to the hospital."

13. The nurse receives a patient post total knee replacement to the surgery. The nurse should prioritize the following, EXCEPT:

    a. Assess for circulation.

    b. Assess for neurologic deficits.

c. Assess for anemia.

d. Assess for bleeding of 2cm on the dressing.

14. A child was brought to the clinic and was diagnosed of having Plumbism. What factor could predispose the child to such disease?

   a. The family travelled to Mexico last summer.

   b. The father's occupation is stained-glass artist.

   c. Their house was built in the year 1977.

   d. The child plays with his brother and sister.

15. A patient status post total hip replacement is ready for discharge. The nurse is preparing a discharge instruction for the patient. Which of the following will help the patient to perform his activities of daily living?

   a. A recliner

   b. A high-seat commode

   c. An abduction pillow

   d. Undergo TENS unit

16. A patient was brought to the emergency room department due to opioid overdose. The nurse should anticipate:

   a. Administration of oxygen via nasal cannula

   b. Naloxone as drug of choice

   c. Cross-matched blood for transfusion

   d. Cardio-resuscitation techniques

17. A patient with irritable bowel syndrome is having abdominal pain, flatus, constipation and diarrhea. Which of the following should the nurse prioritize?

   a. Monitor hydration, intake and output.

   b. Encourage frequent ambulation.

   c. Encourage necessary lifestyle changes to promote stress reduction.

d. Suggest patient to get adequate sleep.

18. A nurse is making room assignments for the day. Which of the following incoming patients should she pair with a 7-year old male patient in Russell's traction due to fractured femur?

   a. A 17-year old female admitted due to therapy for scoliosis.

   b. An 11-year old male for total knee replacement.

   c. A 9-year old male with ALL.

   d. A 5-year old male with osteomyelitis.

19. Pain is one of the most important problems that a nurse should focus on. For a patient with osteoarthritis, the nurse anticipates an order of Celecoxib as the pain medication. What important health teaching should the nurse include?

   a. Take the medication with juice or milk to mask the taste.

   b. Immediately notify the physician for chest pain.

   c. Remain in a sitting position for 30 minutes after taking the medication.

   d. For optimal effect, medication should be taken for 4 weeks.

20. After the surgical repair of tibia, Mark a basketball player, needs the application of Plaster of Paris cast. The nurse should educate Mark on:

   a. How to perform petaling of the cast.

   b. Handling the cast with his fingertips.

   c. Drying the cast with a blower/hair dryer.

   d. Allowing the cast to dry 24 hours before bearing weight.

21. A nurse taking care of a teenage male with a fiberglass cast of his right arm asks the nurse, "Will it be okay if my friends sign my cast?" The nurse should respond:

   a. "Yes, it's okay."

   b. "No, it will weaken the cast."

   c. "Yes, as long as they will not use chalk."

    d. "No, it should remain clear."

22. The nurse doing her rounds saw the LPN doing her pin care for a patient on Skeletal traction. The nurse saw her preparing the things at bedside: sterile gloves, Q-tips, and peroxide. What should the nurse do:

    a. Assist with opening the sterile packages and peroxide.

    b. Change the sterile gloves with clean gloves.

    c. Stop the LPN and tell her she is not allowed to do that.

    d. Tell the LPN to clean the weights and the pulley as well.

23. A patient after several workups was diagnosed of having Multiple Sclerosis. The patient asks the nurse, "What activities should I do away with?" The nurse's response is:

    a. "You should stop with your exercise program."

    b. "You should plan for occupational therapy."

    c. "You should maintain an active lifestyle."

    d. "You should continue personal hygiene."

24. The nurse is taking care of a pediatric patient with a hip dysplasia and has spica cast applied. What nursing intervention is important to prevent side effects of the cast?

    a. Check for the bowel sound.

    b. Assess patient's temperature.

    c. Encourage deep breathing exercises.

    d. Check for the blood pressure.

25. After a total knee replacement, the physician ordered Continuous Passive Machine (CPM) for the patient. The nurse is giving instruction to the patient regarding the machine. Which of the following is the correct information about the machine?

    a. It allows assisted ambulation for the patient.

    b. The controls of the machine are positioned away from the patient.

    c. Pain is a signal to stop the machine.

d. CPM has already a complete therapy and the patient will no longer need therapy after.

26. A patient was brought to the emergency room department with complaints of nausea, vomiting, and abdominal pain. Her friends said that he just started complaining abdominal pain after they eat. The doctor suspects pancreatitis. The nurse should anticipate which diagnostic test?

   a. CBC
   b. Clotting test
   c. X-ray
   d. Serum electrolyte

27. A cardiac patient has an order for routine lab test before her follow-up check-up. In the consulting unit, the doctor noted a serum cholesterol level of 260 mg/dl. The doctor added Rosuvastatin (Crestor) to her medications. The nurse should teach the following, EXCEPT:

   a. Immediately report signs of myopathy, such as muscle weakness.
   b. It should not be taken with antacids.
   c. It should be taken with food.
   d. It should be taken with water.

28. A 36-year old patient with malignant hypertension suddenly exhibited symptoms of hypertensive crisis. The physician ordered stat Diazoxide (Hyperstat) for the patient. Which of the following is the correct nursing intervention with regards to the drug?

   a. Incorporate the drug with D5W and use infusion pump.
   b. Close monitoring of glucose levels.
   c. Position the patient in Trendelenburg position.
   d. Protect the medication with carbon paper/foil.

29. The student nurse is in charge of a 6 year old patient with ventral septal defect receiving Digitalis as part of the child's medication. Which of the following should the student nurse report immediately to the staff nurse?

   a. BP: 110/75 mmHg

   b. Temp: 98°F

   c. HR: 60bpm

   d. RR: 25bpm

30. A 36-year old patient with Peripheral Vascular Disease (PVD) is admitted and being monitored by a nurse. The nurse notes that it is important to assess and monitor the following, EXCEPT:

   a. Distal circulation

   b. Sensory function

   c. Motor function

   d. Pain perception

31. A client is admitted due to right-sided heart failure. The nurse knows that the edema is likely to be found in:

   a. Sacrum

   b. Hands

   c. Neck

   d. Feet

32. The nurse in the ICU unit comes across a doctor's order of measure CVP q 2H. ICU unit come across a doctor's order of measure CVP q 2H. To correctly measure the CVP of the patient, the nurse knows that the zero of the manometer should be aligned with:

   a. Phlebostatic axis

   b. PMI

   c. Erb's point

   d. Tail of Spence

33. A college student was brought to the hospital due edema throughout the body, shortness of breath, flank pain and oliguria. The physician immediately performed a dialysis shunt on the left arm of the patient. Which of the following should NOT be done on the left arm (Note there is more than one Answer)?

   a. Venipuncture.

   b. Blood pressure assessment.

   c. Routine skin care.

   d. Involve in exercise.

34. The nurse is caring for a stroke patient with facial symptoms. Which of the following food should the nurse teach to the family members to prepare?

   a. Iced tea, roast beef, pickles

   b. Pea soup, mashed potatoes, milk

   c. Pumpkin soup, peanut butter and jelly sandwich, tea

   d. Hamburger, fruit salad, coffee

35. One important patient teaching the nurse should give with regards to Novolog is:

   a. It is fast-acting and patient needs to eat after 5-10 minutes of medications.

   b. The patient needs to carry hard candy or some form of sugar all the time.

   c. The patient needs to eat a snack around 2-3 pm.

   d. There is a need for the patient to have a midnight snack.

36. The physician ordered Trimetrexate for a patient diagnosed with leukemia. After a week, the physician placed a new order of Leucovorin calcium to be given to the patient. The nurse should:

   a. Question the order.

   b. Administer the drug.

   c. Mix the drug together.

   d. Alternate the dose of the drug.

37. Mrs. Alonzo brought her 4-month old child in the well-baby clinic for the scheduled immunization. Aside from polio and DPT vaccines, what should the nurse prepare to give the child?

    a. Mumps vaccine

    b. MMR

    c. HibTITER

    d. Hepatitis B vaccine

38. Looking at the patient's chart, the nurse saw new orders for a patient with gastritis. What nursing consideration should the nurse do before administering Esomeprazole?

    a. Advise the patient to take it with meals.

    b. Advise the patient to take it 30 minutes before meals.

    c. Advise the patient to take it at bedtime.

    d. Advise the patient to take it 30 minutes after meals.

39. A patient in the psychiatric unit suddenly burst with rage and shows behavior of aggression and threatening everyone, including the staff. As the charge nurse of the unit, what is the most appropriate action?

    a. Call the security personnel for assistance and prepare to sedate the patient.

    b. Therapeutically talk to the patient to calm down and ask him what game he would like to play.

    c. Call his attention and tell him that a punishment will be given if he continues his bad behavior.

    d. Exclude the patient from the ward activities and ignore him until he calms down.

40. Nurse Lei is doing her rounds to all her postpartum patients. She assesses their fundus and check for signs and complications. One of her patient's fundus is firm, at the level of the umbilicus, but displaced to the right. What is the most appropriate intervention at this time?

    a. Assess for bladder distention.

b. Notify the physician.

c. Assess vital signs, especially blood pressure.

d. Check the signs of bleeding.

41. In the consulting unit, the doctor prescribed Sumatriptan succinate (Imitrex) to the patient with migraine headache. The clinic nurse in charge of explaining the medication should give importance to what symptom to be reported immediately to the doctor?

    a. Angina

    b. Coughing episodes

    c. Diarrhea

    d. Oliguria to anuria

42. There was an ongoing emergency drill in the hospital grounds. One patient is suspected to have a trauma. What method will the nurse utilize to open the airway?

    a. Head tilt

    b. Chin lift

    c. Jaw-thrust

    d. Heimlich

43. The nurse is assisting the physician who is doing an assessment of a patient with suspected Meningitis. The nurse notes that a positive Kernig's sign will show:

    a. Pain when the hip and knee are flexed.

    b. Nuchal rigidity upon flexion of the neck.

    c. Pain when the head is turned to one side.

    d. Feet will flex when arms are extended.

44. The LPN is assisting a patient with Alzheimer's to perform her morning routines. The nurse noted that the patient used her toothbrush for her hair. This is a sign of:

    a. Apraxia

    b. Amnesia

c. Aphasia

d. Agnosia

45. A patient with dementia told the nurse, "What am I doing here?" on one late afternoon. The nurse recognizes that the patient is experiencing:

a. Faulty reasoning

b. Hallucinations

c. Sundowning

d. Agitation

46. In the home care facility, it is time for breakfast for all the patients. After 30 minutes, the nurse went to the hall to check on the seniors. One female patient with Dementia asked the nurse, "When will they bring breakfast?" Which response of the nurse is appropriate?

a. "You already had breakfast 30 minutes ago."

b. "I apologize for the misunderstanding. I'll report it right away."

c. "I'll get you something to eat and drink. What would you like?"

d. "I'm sorry if you didn't have breakfast. You have to wait for lunch."

47. A pediatric patient shows signs of inability to breathe, cough, cry and with bluish lips. The nurse knows that this can be signs of:

a. Cough and colds

b. Vomiting

c. Choking

d. Heart condition

48. In question #47, what is the most effective intervention for the client?

a. CPR

b. Back blows and chest thrusts

c. Chest thrusts

d. Let the patient cough

49. The patient in active labor has a popular lesion on the perineum. What should the nurse do?

    a. Include the assessment in the nurse's notes.

    b. Immediately notify the physician.

    c. Instruct the patient that she will undergo a C-section.

    d. Nothing, just continue with the usual care.

50. A 17-year old primigravida was admitted to the hospital due pain in the upper right side of the abdomen, nausea, vomiting and headache. The physician suspects HELLP. Which of the following is associated with the condition?

    a. Elevated lipoprotein levels

    b. Elevated platelet count

    c. Elevated leukocytes level

    d. Elevated hepatic enzymes

51. A patient in the medical unit suddenly went into cardiac arrest and the nurse started doing CPR, and alerted the code team. The ECG revealed a flat line. How can the nurse confirm if the result is asystole? (NOTE: there is more than one correct answer)

    a. Confirm it in the two leads.

    b. Shock the patient to check the reaction.

    c. Maximize the size of the ECG.

    d. Increase IVF rate.

52. Mrs. Quez a diabetic patient is at 32 weeks AOG. She is scheduled for an amniocentesis to determine the L-S ratio and phosphatidylglycerol levels, hence admitted to the hospital. The result is L-S ratio is 1:1, and presence of phosphatidylglycerol. This assessment shows:

    a. The infant is at high risk of developing heart problems.

b. The infant is at high risk of congenital problems.

c. The infant is at high risk of respiratory problems.

d. The infant is at high risk of birth trauma.

53. The nurse is caring for an infant of a diabetic mother. Which of the following symptoms indicates the need for nursing intervention?

a. Yawning

b. Crying episodes

c. Jitteriness

d. Frequent sleeping

54. A newly assigned staff nurse is caring for a patient with an order of magnesium sulfate IV. The nurse monitors the side effect, which is:

a. Muscle weakness

b. Decrease urine output

c. Hypersomnolence

d. Decrease reflexes

55. A patient with subdural lesion is expected to have increased intracranial pressure. Therefore, the nurse closely monitors the patient for signs of progression of the disease. The nurse noted an abnormal flexion of the patient's body. This condition is known as:

a. Decorticate

b. Decerebrate

c. Neurologic status

d. Cerebral vasoconstriction

56. A pregnant patient opted to have an epidural anesthesia. One of the main side effects is hypotension. What intervention should the nurse perform in case this develops?

a. Position the patient in Trendelenburg

b. Administer oxygen via nasal cannula

c. Administer epinephrine as antidote

d. Increase the rate of the IVF

57. The nurse monitors the patient with ascites. This time a student nurse will handle the patient. To correctly assess for ascites, the student nurse:

    a. Inspect and palpate the abdominal area of the patient.

    b. Tapping the abdomen to observe for "wave" movements.

    c. Measurement of the abdominal girth daily.

    d. Daily weight taking of the patient.

58. A patient was brought to the emergency room department after a motor vehicular accident. Vital signs are taken and as follows: BP-85/30 mmHg, PR-130bpm, RR, 21bpm. Which of the following nursing diagnoses is the priority?

    a. Altered cerebral tissue perfusion

    b. Fluid volume deficit

    c. Ineffective airway clearance

    d. Altered thermoregulation status

59. A nurse is scheduled for a home visit to a 16-year old male diagnosed with osteogenesis imperfecta type 1. During the assessment, what information should cause concern?

    a. Enjoys playing soccer in school.

    b. Frequently drink carbonated drinks during break time.

    c. Has one parent with scoliosis.

    d. He admits taking acetaminophen for pain.

60. A nurse is monitoring a patient having a blood transfusion as treatment for severe anemia. After 5 minutes of the transfusion, the patient complains of pruritus in the chest, arm and burning at the insertion site. The patient also feels chest pain and difficulty of breathing. The nurse notes that these are signs of transfusion reaction. The nurse performs the following:

I. Notify the physician and blood bank of reaction STAT

II. Administer ordered medications

III. Stop the transfusion

IV. Run normal saline to maintain IV access

What is the correct sequence of the interventions?

  a. iii, ii, i, iv

  b. iii, iv, ii, i

  c. iii, iv, i, ii

  d. iii, i, ii, iv

61. A patient with leukemia underwent chemotherapy for treatment. Afterwards, the doctor ordered complete blood count for the patient, which revealed a neutrophil count of 1,500 per microliter of blood. During the visitation, the family brought a fruit basket for the patient. What should the nurse do?

  a. Allow the patient to keep the fruit in her room.

  b. Instruct the patient to place the fruit at the bedside.

  c. Offer to wash the fruits.

  d. Ask the family members to bring the fruit home.

62. In the recovery room, the nurse is taking care of a patient S/P laryngectomy. Upon assessment, the patient looks pale and BP-85/40 mmHg. What should be the most immediate action of the nurse?

  a. Position the patient in Trendelenburg.

  b. Increase the infusion of Normal Saline.

c. Move the emergency cart near the patient.

d. Notify the physician immediately.

63. The patient with a chest tube due to a lung resection accidentally pulls out is tube due to movement. Which intervention by the nurse is appropriate?

a. Notify the physician.

b. Ask the doctor for chest x-ray orders.

c. Attempt to reinsert the tube.

d. Cover the site with Vaseline gauze.

64. The nurse is giving health teaching regarding foods rich in Calcium to a pregnant mother. Which of the following food offers the highest amount of Calcium?

a. Granola Bar

b. Bran muffin

c. Cup of yoghurt

d. Glass of orange juice

65. The nurse is in the community for health teaching, when a child approaches him to go to a place. The nurse saw an elderly whose clothes are soiled with urine and asking for food and water. The nurse knows that the elderly is:

a. Abused

b. Neglected

c. Tired

d. Depressed

66. An 11-year old patient admitted has a hemoglobin count of 10g/dL. The physician orders transfusion of 2 units of blood. The mother did not consent to the blood transfusion and tells the nurse that it is not accepted in their religion. The nurse should:

a. Transfuse the blood if the mother is not there.

b. Encourage the mother the effects of blood transfusion.

c. Teach the consequences of refusal to the treatment.

d. Notify the physician about the refusal.

67. A patient was rushed to the hospital 2 hours after an explosion in his kitchen causes burns to his face and neck. The main priority for the nurse to anticipate to happen is:

a. Hypovolemic shock

b. Laryngeal edema

c. Hyperkalemia

d. Hypernatremia

68. The patient in #67 will be given fluids for his burn. What is the total body surface area affected by burns?

a. 9%

b. 7%

c. 18%

d. 4.5%

69. The nurse in a rehabilitation center is evaluating the improvement of the patient diagnosed with anorexia. Which of the following indicates a positive response to care?

a. "I know the healthy foods from the given menu."

b. "I can cook healthy foods for my family."

c. "My skin improved in color and feel."

d. "My weight increases for about 2lbs."

70. A patient was brought to the emergency room department as the family saw him on the floor. A history revealed that he has abruptly stopped taking in barbiturates. What will the nurse first assess?

a. Signs of depression and suicide intent.

b. Heart rate and diarrhea.

c. Muscle cramps, especially abdominal cramps.

d. Euphoria and tachycardia.

71. The nurse is assessing a laboring patient. The nurse notes that the FHT is loudest in the upper-left quadrant. What position of the infant will the nurse suspect?

   a. Right breech presentation.

   b. Left occipital transverse presentation.

   c. Right occipital anterior presentation.

   d. Left sacral anterior presentation.

72. The nurse observed that one of her patients diagnosed with manic disorder was unable to finish her breakfast. What should the nurse do to help her have adequate nutrition?

   a. Always serve the patient high-calorie foods that she can carry anywhere.

   b. Join her during breakfast to monitor her intake and encourage her to eat.

   c. Serve her small portions of food presented in an attractive way.

   d. Instruct her to list down the different food she wants to have.

73. The nurse is giving a presentation to her co-nurses in the hospital regarding burns. The topic is TBSA (total body surface area). The nurse said that in order to approximate the percentage of an area, the measurement depends on:

   a. The thumb as 1%

   b. Four finger beds as 1%

   c. One palm as 1%

   d. One fist as 1%

74. The nurse is taking care of a patient with herpes lesion. Which action of the nurse shows understanding of the condition?

   a. Proper wound dressing techniques in covering the wound.

   b. The use of gloves in caring for the patient.

   c. The nurse should administer all the prescribed medications.

   d. The nurse should limit visitors.

75. The physician ordered a trough for a patient receiving 5 doses of Vancomycin infusion. When is the most appropriate time to collect the sample for the trough?

    a. 30 minutes after the infusion

    b. 30 minutes before the infusion.

    c. 1 hour after the infusion.

    d. 1 hour before the infusion.

76. The patient in the family planning unit is asking the nurse how to use the diaphragm. Which of the following is the correct information about diaphragm?

    a. Do not keep the diaphragm in for no longer than 5 hours.

    b. The diaphragm should be placed in a cool place.

    c. The diaphragm should be changed every 6 months.

    d. The diaphragm has a universal size.

77. The nurse asked the student nurse regarding the symptom of damage to Cranial Nerve VII. Which of the following is the most appropriate response?

    a. "I should be able to assess facial pain."

    b. "The patient should complain of inability to smell."

    c. "I will be able to observe no eye movement."

    d. "The patient will have difficulty in swallowing."

78. A child was seen in the bathtub unconscious and was rushed to the hospital. An immediate response to revive the child was initiated by the medical team. One cause of this incident that the nurse should consider is:

    a. The child is playful.

    b. The child is hiding from the parents.

    c. The child does not know how to swim.

    d. The child is abused.

79. A patient with urinary tract infection is given Phenazopyridine hydrochloride (Pyridium). The nurse should teach the patient about:

   a. It is an antibiotic and should be taken after meals.

   b. It is an analgesic and may change the color of your urine.

   c. It is an antipyretic and can cause diarrhea.

   d. It is a diuretic and pruritus as the common side effect.

80. The nurse should question a doctor's order of Accutane for a patient who is:

   a. Having diarrhea.

   b. Pregnant.

   c. Has a heart problem.

   d. Has an allergy to seafood.

81. The nurse is teaching an AIDS patient regarding Acyclovir. Which of the following are the correct patient teachings:

   I. Acyclovir can be taken with or without food.

   II. Acyclovir should not be taken if you're feeling better.

   III. It should be taken with a full glass of water.

   IV. You should perform ADLs with caution.

   a. i, ii, iii

   b. i, ii, iv

   c. i, iii, iv

   d. ii, iii, iv

82. A patient will need to undergo MRI as part of diagnostic test. She told the nurse that she is 4 weeks pregnant and is afraid that MRI will cause damage to her child. The nurse should:

   a. Notify the physician immediately.

   b. Explain to the patient that it is okay to undergo the procedure.

   c. Halt the procedure and opt to another diagnostic procedure.

d. Let the patient sign in the chart for refusal.

83. A patient was admitted to the hospital due to the following symptoms: 102°F, profuse sweating, fatigue, headache and agitation, tachypnea, and tachycardia. The nurse notes that this kind of hyperthermia is:

a. Heat edema

b. Heat syncope

c. Heat exhaustion

d. Heat stroke

84. The nurse is scheduled for a home visit to the following patients. Which should she visit first?

a. A diabetic patient with glucose level of 90mg/dL.

b. A hypertensive patient eating homemade pasta.

c. A patient with chest pain and a history of angina.

d. An AIDS patient maintained on Acyclovir.

85. A 34-year old patient was diagnosed with cystic fibrosis and was given pancreatic enzyme supplements. As part of the educating the client, the nurse should:

a. Instruct the patient to take it once in the morning after breakfast.

b. Instruct him to take the medication 3 times a day, 1 hour prior each meal.

c. Instruct him to take the medication 3 times a day with meal.

d. Instruct him to take it once before bedtime.

86. The patient will undergo tests to determine cataract. The nurse knows that cataract affects the lens which:

a. Controls the stimulation of the retina.

b. Coordinates eye movement.

c. Focuses the light rays on the retina.

d. Magnifies small objects.

87. One of the eyedrops given to a patient with glaucoma is miotic agents. The nurse knows that miotic agents:

    a. Reduce pressure in the eye.

    b. Dilate the pupils.

    c. Constrict the pupils.

    d. Reduce the production of fluid.

88. A patient diagnosed with severe corneal ulcer has a prescription of Gentamycin drop every 4hours and Neomycin drop every 4hours. How will the nurse administer the medications to the patient?

    a. Administer the first medication and the second after 5 minutes.

    b. Administer the first and the second one after the other.

    c. Administer separately using cycloplegic eye drop.

    d. Question the order of the patient.

89. A patient arrived in the emergency room department due to frostbite injury. Which of the following interventions should NOT be done by the nurse?

    a. Cover the infected part with loose, dry, sterile bandage.

    b. Soak the area in warm water.

    c. Rub the affected area and pop the blisters.

    d. Separate frostbitten toes and fingers with sterile gauze.

90. A patient diagnosed with color blindness asked the nurse the color that she will most likely have difficulty seeing. The nurse responds:

    a. "You will only be able to see black and white."

    b. "You will not see reds and orange."

    c. "You will not be able to see blues and violets."

    d. "You will have difficulty seeing yellow."

91. A patient with a pacemaker is ready for discharge. As part of discharge instructions, the nurse should put attention to:

   a. Notify the physician if there is a headache.

   b. Monitor blood pressure daily.

   c. Do not use electronic appliances that have radiation, such as a microwave oven.

   d. Daily monitoring of pulse rate.

92. The nurse is teaching a mother of a 6-year old patient with enuresis. She asked the nurse, "What if my son asks for a drink at night after we had dinner, what should I do?" The nurse's best response is:

   a. "Do not give anymore, and tell him that fluid is not good at night."

   b. "Give him just a spoon of water."

   c. "Give him water 2 hours before sleep."

   d. "Just a few sips of fluid is okay before sleeping."

93. A 22-year old woman asks the nurse about what food should she have to help prevent recurrence of UTI. The nurse knows that alkaline foods can help the patient. Which of the following should the nurse recommend?

   a. Fresh vegetable salad with apple cider dressing.

   b. Increase intake of orange, mango and grape juice.

   c. Serve corned beef or turkey meat for breakfast.

   d. Drink a glass of cranberry juice daily.

94. A diabetic patient in the outpatient department is listening to the nurse while giving patient teaching regarding NPH. Which of the following responses of the patient shows understanding?

   a. "I will use NPH after I eat breakfast."

   b. "I will eat breakfast after 2 hours of injecting NPH."

   c. "I will eat something at around 3-4 pm."

   d. "I need to have a meal between dinner and breakfast."

95. The nurse checks the patient's chart regarding the some medications; she then checked the ampule of the medication. Which of the following should she check?

    a. The quantity, the name, and the dosage.

    b. The expiration date, strength and route.

    c. The label, the expiration date and manufacturing date.

    d. The unit of measure, the availability in the pharmacy, and the brand.

96. During the rounds, a postpartum mother tells the nurse that she plans to breastfeed her child. The nurse knows that for breastfeeding to be successful depends most on:

    a. The mother's ability to carry the child.

    b. The infant's birth weight.

    c. The size of the mother's breast.

    d. The mother's desire to breastfeed.

97. Nurse Lena is in charge of monitoring a 31-year old pregnant mother's progress of labor. Which of the following assessment should she report immediately to the physician?

    a. Uterine contractions radiating to the back and relieved by walking.

    b. Complaints of the patient having to urinate frequently.

    c. A discharge that shows a green-tinged amniotic fluid.

    d. The presence of scanty bloody discharge.

98. The nurse will measure the duration of contraction of a patient in labor. Which of the following describes the correct method of measurement?

    a. It is measured from the beginning of one contraction to the beginning of the next contraction.

    b. It is measured from the end of one contraction to the beginning of the next contraction.

    c. It is measured from the beginning of one contraction to the end of that contraction.

    d. It is measured from the end of one contraction to the end of the next contraction.

99. The doctor called with new orders for a particular patient. In order to prevent medication errors the nurse writes down the order in the doctor's notes and:

    a. Write them using medical abbreviations that can be understood by all.

    b. Write them in a legible manner.

    c. Write them word per word, including word fillers.

    d. Write them without abbreviations and symbols.

100. A pregnant diabetic patient at 26 weeks AOG, visits the prenatal clinic. The patient is wondering why the doctor prescribed her a higher dose of insulin. Which of the following statement describes the role of insulin in pregnancy? (NOTE: more than one answer is correct.)

    a. Insulin requirement increases as the pregnancy progresses.

    b. Insulin requirement is moderated as the pregnancy progresses.

    c. Insulin requirement starts high, but decreases as pregnancy progresses.

    d. Fetal development depends on the adequate regulation of insulin.

ANSWERS:

1. Correct Answer: B.

The signs point directly to a Congestive Heart Failure. And to determine if it is right-sided or left-sided, here is the clue: left-sided is pulmonary based, while right sided is vascular based.

2. Correct Answer: C.

A newborn with the narcotic abstinence syndrome is easily irritable therefore comfort with decrease stimulus is needed for the baby. Choices A and D will make the child irritable. Choice B is still inappropriate for the newborn.

3. Correct Answer: A.

One of the side effects of epidural anesthesia is hypotension that if not monitored will result in shock. The patient should be monitored every 15 minutes to secure that this will not happen. Choice B and C can be done once the patient is stable. Choice D is dangerous as the anesthesia can travel to the respiratory center.

4. Correct Answer: B.

Hand washing is the number one way of preventing infection and cross-contamination in any cases. Choice A and C are correct measures, but are less effective than hand washing. Choice D is incorrect as post-operative patients need frequent monitoring.

5. Correct Answer: B.

There are two main types of Diabetes: Type 1 and Type 2. Type 1 results from a primary failure of pancreatic beta cells to produce insulin. Type 2 results from the development of insulin resistance in body cells. And it is considered as a chronic metabolic disorder marked by hyperglycemia.

6. Correct Answer: B.

A noticeable misalignment of the hip with the extremity should be noted. Choice A is incorrect as all fractures do have pain. Choices C and D indicates different diseases, such compartment syndrome and PVD.

7. Correct Answer: B.

During menopause the women also decrease the amount of hormones in their body, one of which is responsible in absorbing and utilizing calcium in the body. Choice A is wrong as lack of exercise in not the main cause. Choice C is done to prevent osteoporosis, but not because serum calcium decreases. Choice D is wrong as it is not inherited.

8. Correct Answer: B.

In Bryant's traction, the pull starts from the buttocks and there are no pins (this is found in Skeletal traction). Note that the extremities (both the left and the right legs are suspended in the traction at a ninety degree angle with the knees slightly flexed). Also Bryant's traction is the choice for pediatric clients.

9. Correct Answer: B.

For optimum bone healing and bone alignment, traction is needed to reduce pain, muscle spasms, which can disrupt bone alignment. It will also restore the alignment of the bones as they heal. And prevents hip flexion contractures and pressure sores.

10. Correct Answer: D.

Most especially considering the part involved, hemorrhage should always be assessed as this is the most life-threatening complication of surgery. Pain will be present and is controlled by medications. Nutritional intake is not yet necessary as this is post-surgery, and nutrients come from the IVF first, until she is ready to eat. Physical therapy will come at a later stage.

11. Correct Answer: B.

They should not jump into conclusion in agreeing that the patient has hypertension. Hypertension is a persistence of the intermittent elevation of systolic BP greater that 140mmHg or diastolic BP greater than 90mmHg. Therefore, the nurse should assess further to know what is the normal BP, or the usual BP that the client has.

12. Correct Answer: A.

The wife and the family members should be taught on how to feed the patient properly. One important technique is flushing the tube after feeding and not to forget to clamp it. Choice B should be done before feeding, not at any time of the day. Choice C should not cause an alarm, as it can be treated with medications. Choice D is inappropriate as the patient will not swallow the food.

13. Correct Answer: D.

The nurse should check for circulation by capillary refill, warmth, color and pedal pulses. The nurse should also check dorsiflexion, plantar flexion and toe wiggling for signs of neurologic deficits. And anemia reflected in the hematocrit count of the patient. However, a bleeding of 2cm on the dressing is considered normal.

14. Correct Answer: B.

Plumbism is actually lead poisoning. This has several factors such as using a pottery from Central America or Mexico in cooking, so just travelling will not cause it; the house is built in 1975 or lower years, because lead was removed from paint in 1976; it is not genetic; and there is somebody who, mostly the parent, who are skilled stained-glass artist.

15. Correct Answer: B.

To help in the healing process, the hips should be kept higher than the knees of the patient. Looking at the given choices, the high-seat commode keeps the knees, lower than the hips and help with activities of daily livings.

16. Correct Answer: B.

Naloxone is the drug of choice for narcotic and anesthesia overdose. The nurse should anticipate the prescription of Naloxone as the immediate intervention for the patient. If the patient is hypoxic then oxygen should be administered by mask. There is no need to perform choices C and D.

17. Correct Answer: A.

Following The Maslow's Hierarchy of needs the patient's nutrition should be monitored, especially the patient is having abdominal problems.

18. Correct Answer: B.

In order to pick the best person to be a roommate to the given client, the first rule is the same gender. Therefore, choice A is incorrect. Next, is to check the condition of the different patients, choice C is immunocompromised, choice D has an infection. Therefore the safest is choice B, closest in age and with similarity in the case of the 7-year old.

19. Correct Answer: B.

Celecoxib is a COX-2 inhibitor medication. This group of drugs was associated with heart attack and stroke. Part of the teaching should include signs and symptoms related to heart problems (chest pain), and abdominal symptoms (black/tarry stools).

20. Correct Answer: D.

Plaster of Paris cast should be allowed to dry for 24 hours. This will ensure that it is equally dried and will not break before bearing weight. After it dries, then the nurse can now teach the patient to do choice A. Fingertips will not offer the best support, the whole palm should be used. Choice C will cause unequal drying and burn on the patient's casted part.

21. Correct Answer: A.

There is no proof that marker pens will do harm on the cast. Therefore, it is okay to let his friends sign on it.

22. Correct Answer: A.

The LPN is qualified to clean the Steinmann pins as long as she follows the sterile techniques. Since the LPN is ready, the nurse can just assist the LPN with the opening the sterile packs. And there is no need to clean the weights and the pulley.

23. Correct Answer: C.

The goal of therapy for patients with Multiple Sclerosis is to control the symptoms and preserve function to maximize quality of life. The nurse should encourage healthful and active lifestyle to maintain good muscle tone, good nutrition, and plenty of rest and relaxation.

24. Correct Answer: A.

A spica cast is also known as a body cast that starts from the abdomen to the legs/knees (at times until the foot of the patient, depending on the case). The most common side effect is paralytic ileus, and the nurse should assess for the bowel sounds. Choice B, C, and D do not address the side effect.

25. Correct Answer: B.

Pain should be expected during the therapy, but it should not be a reason to stop the machine. The patient will not be able to ambulate, CPM is an in bed therapy. After hospitalization, the patient is encouraged to have physical therapy. The controls should be positioned away from the patient so that he will not be able to manipulate the controls or turn it off when there is pain.

26. Correct Answer: D.

Pancreatitis is diagnosed by the following tests: pancreatic function test to assess the production of digestive enzymes; Glucose tolerance test to measure damage to cells producing insulin; Ultrasound or CT scan to assess pancreas; blood tests such as serum glucose, electrolyte test for Ca, Mg, Na, and potassium, as well as bicarbonate levels.

27. Correct Answer: C.

Rosuvastatin is an antilipemic, HMG-COA reductase inhibitor and prescribed for increased serum cholesterol (normal: <200 mg/dl). The nurse should teach choices A, B and C. It should be taken 2 hours before or after antacids, it can be taken with or without food, and only with water as it interacts with juice.

28. Correct Answer: B.

Diazoxide is an anti-hypertensive, vasodilator, and cardiovascular agent given intravenously to patient for emergency lowering of BP. The common side effect is hyperglycemia, therefore close monitoring of blood glucose is important, as well as BP for the first 15 to 30 minutes after administration. The patient should be placed in a Dorsal Recumbent position to decrease the work load of the heart. And it does not react with light; therefore, there is no need to cover.

29. Correct Answer: C.

Digitalis is given to the patient to make the heart muscles stronger and regulate the heartbeat. Choices A, B and D are incorrect as they will not show the effect of the medication, and they are in the normal range. Choice C is not normal, as the dose should already be withheld if the HR is <100bpm.

30. Correct Answer: D.

Pain in PVD is relieved by rest and the patient is given medication for its alleviation. The nurse should now focus on the progression of the disease by assessing and monitoring choice A, B and C.

31. Correct Answer: C.

This is known as Jugular Vein Distention (JVD) and the most apparent sign of right-sided heart failure.

32. Correct Answer: A.

The phlebostatic axis is located at the fourth intercostal space midaxillary line or mid-anterior-posterior chest wall. This is the location of the right atrium. Choice B is at 5th ICS Midclavicular line. Choice C is on the 3rd ICS left sternal border; this is where S2 is best heard (auscultated). Choice D is part of the breast where cancer cells are mostly seen.

33. Correct Answer: A and B.

The left hand of the patient has a shunt used for dialysis, if pressure is placed on the arm (BP taking) as it will burst the vein involved. The blood taken in the area is also not suitable as a sample to be analyzed. However, choice C is okay to promote health. Choice D as long as no pressure is placed on the arm, such as arm raising and swaying is alright.

34. Correct Answer: B.

A stroke patient with facial symptoms has a difficulty of chewing and swallowing. Therefore, the food choice should be easily swallowed and will need less chewing, making choice B the perfect choice.

35. Correct Answer: A.

Novolog is a kind of fast-acting insulin that works by lowering the levels of blood sugar. Therefore, the patient needs to eat again within 5-10 minutes.

36. Correct Answer: B.

The nurse should administer the drug, Leucovorin calcium is given to counteract the toxicity of Trimetrexate in the patient. Therefore, choices A, C, and D are incorrect.

37. Correct Answer: C.

The 4-month old child should receive the following standard vaccines: DPT (or DTaP), IPV (Polio vaccine), RV (Rotavirus vaccine), PCV (Pneumococcal vaccine), and HibTITER. Choice A and B are given at 12 months. Choice D was given at birth and given within 1-2 months and 6-18 months.

38. Correct Answer: A.

Esomeprazole is classified under proton pump inhibitors, which should be taken with meals. Most H2 antagonists should be taken 30 minutes before meals, such as Zantac. However, Tagamet, also an H2 antagonist medication is taken as a single dose at bedtime. Choice D does not describe gastric medications.

39. Correct Answer: A.

The patient behavior is already dangerous to him and to the staff, and needs restraint of the security and sedation by the nurses. Choice B won't work, as the patient's aggression will not let him listen. Choice C will only make the situation worse, because of the punishment. Choice D will not solve the problem; it will continue and might be risky to the staff.

40. Correct Answer: A.

The fundus should be found at the center and slowly going back to its normal state. However, displacement to the side indicates full bladder. The nurse should catheterize the patient next.

41. Correct Answer: A.

Angina, chest pain, feelings of heaviness, pressure or tightness should be reported immediately to the doctor. The nurse should teach the side effects of the patient and learn the history, as it should not be given to patients with a history of heart attack, cardiovascular problems, smoking, allergies to sulphonamides, and seizure.

42. Correct Answer: C.

Jaw thrust is recommended for all ages that is suspected with trauma. Choices A and B go together if the patient has no trauma. Choice D is an intervention for airway obstruction.

43. Correct Answer: A.

A positive Kernig's sign is when there is pain on the flexion of the hip and the knee. Nuchal rigidity will not allow the neck to flex forward. Choice C and D do not pertain to Meningitis assessment.

44. Correct Answer: A.

Here are the five As of Alzheimer's Disease: Apraxia refers to the inability to use objects because of failure to identify them; Amnesia is memory loss; Aphasia is inability to express oneself through speech; Agnosia is the inability to recognize familiar objects, and other sensations; and Anomia is the inability to remember the names of things.

45. Correct Answer: C.

Sundowning refers to the patients increased confusion during the night. Choice A, B and D are all symptoms of dementia, but is not related to confusions in the afternoon.

46. Correct Answer: C.

The nurse should accept some of the reality of the patient with Dementia, especially if it will not harm in any way. In the case, the patient forgot the intake of food, therefore the nurse should accept it. Arguing will not lead to the solution of the problem. It will not satisfy the patient, so getting what she needs will make her feel comfortable.

47. Correct Answer: C.

Here are the different signs of choking in babies: bluish skin color, difficulty in breathing, inability to cry or make sounds, weak or ineffective coughing, and soft or high-pitched sound in inspiration.

48. Correct Answer: B.

For infants, the best intervention is alternate five back flows and five chest thrusts until the obstruction relieved or unresponsiveness occurs. Choice A is used for adults and infants who are unconscious.

49. Correct Answer: B.

A lesion in the perineum can point towards herpes, or an infection. If it is an open wound, the patient will need to deliver via C-section. Choice A and D are incorrect as this finding is significant to the health of the child. Choice C needs a doctor's order and not a decision the nurse should do.

50. Correct Answer: D.

HELLP stands for Hemolysis, Elevated Liver enzymes, Low Platelet count. Therefore choices A, B and C are not related to HELLP.

51. Correct Answer: A and C.

To rule out other ECG reading such as atrial fibrillation or PEA, the size of the ECG should be maximized. Also, two leads should confirm the flat line or asystole before CPR is no longer done. Choice B will create reaction to the patient, but will not confirm asystole. Choice D will not affect ECG results.

52. Correct Answer: C.

L-S stands for Lecithin-Salphingomyelin ratio and indicates fetal lung maturity. A ratio of 2 or more means maturity of the fetal lung and decreases the risk of respiratory distress syndrome. It is not related to choices A, B, and D.

53. Correct Answer: C.

Jitteriness for the infant is a sign of seizure. Choices A, B, and D are actually normal activities by the infant.

54. Correct Answer: C.

The common side effects of magnesium include: confusion, dizziness, and sleepiness (Hypersomnolence). Choice A, B, and D are signs of magnesium sulfate toxicity.

55. Correct Answer: A.

Decorticate is the abnormal flexion of the extremities of a patient with ICP. Decerebrate is an abnormal extension. Choices C and D are factors needed for collaborative management of a patient with ICP.

56. Correct Answer: D.

If the patient develops hypotension, increasing the BP until it reaches the normal range is the main priority. Interventions include positioning the patient in recumbent/side lying position – trendelenburg will cause the anesthesia to travel to the respiratory center; oxygen via mask, not nasal cannula; increasing IVF infusion. If measures do not provide changes, notify the physician, and prepare epinephrine at bedside.

57. Correct Answer: C.

Although choice D provides objective data, it does not reflect ascites alone. Therefore, choice C mainly targets the abdomen. Using a paper tape measure and marking the same spot to be measured will determine changes in the abdomen. Choices A and B are also pertaining to assessment of the abdomen, however, they are more subjective.

58. Correct Answer: B.

The given vital signs are an indication of hypovolemic shock. Therefore, increasing the circulating blood and fluid in the patient's body is the main priority. Choices A, C, and D might be diagnosed in the latter stages, but not a main priority.

59. Correct Answer: A.

Osteogenesis imperfecta is a genetic disorder characterized having bones that break easily. Therefore, physical activities, such as sports and exercise can actually promote fracture to the patient. Choices B, C, and D does not cause alarm for the patient.

60. Correct Answer: C.

The correct order is to stop the transfusion first and run the normal saline solution to maintain the IV access. Notify the physician and the blood bank of the reaction STAT. Recheck patient ID and blood labels for possible errors. Return unused blood product to the blood bank for analysis. And administer ordered medications immediately.

61. Correct Answer: D.

A patient with decreased neutrophil count (neutropenia) is at risk for infection. Therefore, part of teaching is for the family not to bring anything fresh for the patient. This includes fruits and flowers.

62. Correct Answer: B.

The most immediate action is to increase the infusion of Normal Saline in order to prevent further hypotension. Choice A is dangerous since the patient had a neck surgery. The position can cause further obstruction of the airway. Choice C is not necessary at the moment. Choice D is done after nursing interventions are done.

63. Correct Answer: D.

Vaseline gauze is an occlusive dressing used to cover the insertion site. This is necessary to help the lungs function well in a closed system, before reporting to the doctor what happen. Do not attempt to reinsert the tube.

64. Correct Answer: C.

The best source of Calcium is dairy products, such as milk and cheese. Among the choices, yoghurt is the only milk product. Choices A, B and D have some calcium in them.

65. Correct Answer: B.

Malnutrition, dehydration, poor hygiene are signs of elderly neglect. If restraints are present, then it's abused. Choices C and D are inappropriate choices.

66. Correct Answer: D.

The refusal should be noted and signed by the mother in the chart. The physician should be notified to talk to the mother about other possible treatment for the child, since the patient is still a minor. In some cases, a court order is needed for the treatment. These make choices A, B, and C incorrect.

67. Correct Answer: B.

One complication of burns in the face, neck and chest is airway obstruction due to laryngeal edema. The next priority is hypovolemia that can lead to shock if untreated. The last priority should be electrolyte imbalance as well as the arterial blood gases.

68. Correct Answer: D.

The head is accounted for 4.5% for TBSA (total body surface area). Legs are considered 9% each. 7% are the TBSA for the legs of an infant. 18% is the chest of the adult.

69. Correct Answer: D.

The best indicator is an objective data, such as the weight of the patient. The nurse should monitor the weight of the patient to check if the plan of care is effective. Choice A and B are not enough, as it only shows her knowledge. Choice C is an effect of healthy food; however, it does not show that the patient is able to fight against anorexia.

70. Correct Answer: B.

Barbiturates becomes the go to drug for some people who want to have stress relief and experiencing insomnia as the medication creates a sedative effect. If stopped abruptly, it can cause hyperthermia, abdominal problems and circulatory problems (tachycardia). Therefore, choice B shows what the nurse should be assessing for.

71. Correct Answer: D.

If the position of the fetus is in the Left sacral anterior presentation, the fetal heart tones will be heard in the upper left quadrant. If the heart tones are in the right upper quadrant, the choice is A. If the heart tones are in the left lower quadrant the fetus is in the choice B presentation. If the heart tones are in the right lower quadrant it would be choice C.

72. Correct Answer: A.

A Manic patient is described as having an elevated mood, they can be cheerful and euphoric, but at times irritable. It is difficult for them to sit down or maintain a position for a very long time. Therefore the nurse should focus on giving the patient high-caloric diet on the go. It would be very difficult for the nurse to perform choice B because of the problem of attention. Choice C is good, but will not offer good nutrition needed by the manic patient. Choice D will also be difficult to attain, and listing down will not provide the nutrition she needs.

73. Correct Answer: C.

TBSA is based on the palm of one hand that is equal to approximately 1%. This is the standard used to measure TBSA not the thumb, fingers or the fist.

74. Correct Answer: B.

A patient with herpes lesion or herpes zoster should be placed in contact precaution. Therefore the nurse should protect herself in caring for the patient, such as wearing gloves in caring for the patient. It is not necessary to do choice A, there are no antibiotics prescribed and the nurse should teach about contact precaution to the family relatives.

75. Correct Answer: B.

The rule getting a sample for the trough is to get it 30 minutes before the infusion of the medication, preferably before the 3rd or the 4th dose. If done after the infusion, the sample will not be reliable in checking the effectiveness of the patient. One hour is too long.

76. Correct Answer: B.

In taking care of the diaphragm it should be placed in a cool place. It can be placed inside the woman for longer than 6 hours. If cleaned properly, it can last up to 2 years. The diaphragm has no universal size; it should be fitted to the woman.

77. Correct Answer: A.

Cranial nerve VII is Facial nerve. Therefore the answer should be related to facial movement and pain. Choice B is olfactory nerve (CN I). Choice C is oculomotor nerve (CN III). Choice D is glossopharyngeal nerve (CN IX).

78. Correct Answer: D.

Drowning or near drowning situations for the child, especially in bathtubs and bucket is associated with child abuse. Therefore, choices A, B, and C are incorrect.

79. Correct Answer: B.

It is an analgesic used to relieve pain in UTI, but not to treat the infection. The nurse should teach that the patient should not be alarmed if her urine changes color (orange to red). It is not an antibiotic, antipyretic or a diuretic.

80. Correct Answer: B.

Accutane or isotretinoin is a medication used to treat acne. It is teratogenic to pregnant women, therefore for women using this, a pregnancy test is important. It is not contraindicated in patients in choices A, C, and D.

81. Correct Answer: C.

Acyclovir treatment can be taken with no regards to food, and should be with a full glass of water. During the treatment, it is encouraged that the patient increases the amount of fluid taken in. Common side effects are dizziness, headache and nausea; therefore, a need for caution in doing ADLs. However, it should be taken for the prescribed duration, even if already feeling well.

82. Correct Answer: B.

The Safety Committee of the Society of Magnetic Resonance Imaging supports the notion of using MRI to pregnant women if the need arises and no other examination can be done. The physician or the nurse should tell that up to this date, MRI has no significant effect on a pregnant patient based on clinical studies. An example of the need is if there is a suspected fetal anomaly or disorder.

83. Correct Answer: C.

Heat exhaustion happens when the patient's body is getting warm or hot. He becomes thirsty, weak, the temperature is less than 104°F, and is due to depletion of salt and water in the body. Choice A is edema or swelling in the feet when it is hot. Choice B is sudden unconsciousness after physical activity under the heat. And choice D is temperature higher than 104°F, unconsciousness, absence of sweat, and many other signs that are life threatening.

84. Correct Answer: C.

A patient with chest pain is at risk of myocardial infarction and therefore needs the utmost attention of the nurse. Choice A's glucose level is within normal range. Choice B means that the patient is changing his lifestyle. And choice D does not pose any threat to his health.

85. Correct Answer: C.

A patient with cystic fibrosis will need to drink supplements such as pancreatic enzymes for as long as the disease is with him. It should be taken three times a day with meals for it to take effect in digesting the food ingested by the patient, making the other choices incorrect.

86. Correct Answer: C.

The lens is the part of the eye found behind the iris that bends the light rays in order to form a clear image at the back of the eye.

87. Correct Answer: C.

Miotic or cholinergic agents increase the outflow of fluid in the eye. It does this by constricting the pupils. Betablockers do choice A. They do not dilate the pupils. And carbonic anhydrase inhibitors do choice D.

88. Correct Answer: A.

The nurse should always give time to allow the eye drops to be absorbed first before the other one. The minimum time is 5 minutes. Choices A and D are incorrect and the medications can be administered together. Choice C is not necessary.

89. Correct Answer: C.

It would be dangerous to rub the affected area as it can be the cause of removing that part from the body. Popping the blisters will only cause wound as the area will not be able to heal. Choices A, B, and D are correct interventions.

90. Correct Answer: C.

Patients with color blindness will actually have problems in distinguishing the shades of color blue, violet and green.

91. Correct Answer: D.

The patient with a pacemaker should be instructed to monitor and record his pulse rate daily, since the pacemaker is placed on his heart. Choice A is not necessary. Choice B is okay to monitor blood pressure and effectiveness of medication. Choice C is okay as long as the patient stands 5 feet away when it is on.

Kaye

92. Correct Answer: C.

The nurse should reiterate to the mother to be strict in implementing the home plan to train the bladder of the child. The most sensible plan is to give a glass or half a glass of water to the child 2-3 hours before sleeping, so that there will be a chance for him to urinate before sleeping.

93. Correct Answer: D.

Among the choices, only the cranberry juice is considered as alkaline. Choices A, B, and C are acidic foods.

94. Correct Answer: C.

NPH has a shorter action with a peak time of 4-9 hours, showing the larger duration. Therefore, if NPH is given at breakfast, the patient needs to eat a snack at around 3 to 4 pm.

95. Correct Answer: B.

Although all the following is important in checking the drug, there are actually some incorrect things per choice. In choice A, the nurse shouldn't check the dosage on the label; it depends on the physician's order. Choice C, there is no need to check the manufacturing date. And choice D, the availability in the pharmacy makes it incorrect.

96. Correct Answer: D.

There are many factors for breastfeeding to be successful, however the other factors will not be successful if the mother has no desire to breastfeed the child. Choices A, B, C and D are not important in breastfeeding.

97. Correct Answer: C.

This shows signs of meconium staining, which is dangerous to the fetus. Choice A is false labor. Choice B and D are normal.

98. Correct Answer: C.

Duration of contraction refers to how long one contraction is. It should be timed from the beginning of one contraction until it ends. Choice A, B and D shows two contractions, making them incorrect.

99. Correct Answer: D.

The nurse should write in a legible manner, however, it is full of abbreviations and symbols, it can cause medication errors. Therefore, the nurse should put choice D first more than anything else.

100. Correct Answer: A and D.

The fetal development depends on the adequacy and regulation of insulin and nutrition. As pregnancy progresses, the insulin intake increases, depending on the physician's assessment of the patient (and the fetus).

IV. NCLEX Exam Four

QUESTIONS:

1. The nurse is missing Humalog and Regular insulin. To ensure that medication errors be avoided, the nurse should:

    a. Read the order again and place the chart in front while mixing.

    b. Draw them in different syringes before mixing them in a medicine cup.

    c. Have a second nurse as a witness and double check the dose and type.

    d. Mix the insulin while the physician is observing.

2. A patient was brought to the emergency room department with complaints of chest pain. The family member said that they were just watching and suddenly his father complains of pain. What intervention should the nurse perform first?

    a. Perform an ECG.

b. Auscultate the patient's chest.

c. Assess vital signs.

d. Interview to gather history.

3. A nurse is caring for an American-Chinese patient in the terminal stages of liver cancer. The family and the relatives of the patient brought in some incense and wore their traditional clothes. What should the nurse do?

a. Set a limit on the visiting hours and ask the family to bring the incense home.

b. Notify the family that they need to do their rituals at home.

c. Provide policy for the family and comfort the family.

d. Tell the family that it is against hospital policy.

4. The charge nurse is making the staff assignments for the day. A floater was sent from the labor unit to be part of the team of the cardiac unit for this day. Which patient should the floater handle?

a. A patient status post coronary bypass, a week ago, ready for discharge.

b. A patient for an angiogram and is suspected with myocardial infarction monitored on telemetry.

c. A patient diagnosed with unstable angina in need of close monitoring.

d. A patient status post valve replacement admitted to the unit.

5. A mother of a newly-diagnosed 6-year old child with diabetes mellitus type 1 is receiving discharge instructions. The mother asks the nurse, "What is Glucagon for?" The nurse responds based on the knowledge that Glucagon:

a. Augments the effects of insulin in cases where insulin seems not working after an hour.

b. Treats hypoglycemia in cases of insulin overdose.

c. Treats the side effect of injecting insulin, which is lipoatrophy.

d. It lengthens the effect of insulin, therefore, decreases the insulin injection.

6. A patient admitted due to vomiting and diarrhea. The nurse should anticipate what IV solution?

    a. 0.9% NaCl

    b. D5W

    c. D5NS

    d. LR

7. A pediatric patient diagnosed with congestive heart failure is receiving Furosemide therapy. The nurse should teach the mother of the patient to report:

    a. A sudden weight gain.

    b. A decrease in blood pressure.

    c. An increase in feeding.

    d. A slow heart rate.

8. A patient receiving Phenytoin for seizure is having breakthrough seizures. The nurse notified the physician, which in turn ordered for a blood sample to be withdrawn. Which of the following indicate ineffectiveness of the drug?

    a. 19 mcg/ml

    b. 5 mcg/ml

    c. 15 mcg/ml

    d. 10 mcg/ml

9. A 26-year old patient was brought to the emergency room department due to abdominal pain radiating to the back. A history reveals that the patient has taken 2 acetaminophen tablets every three hours for headache and does not give relief. The doctor suspects toxicity which can be confirmed by:

    a. Hearing test.

    b. Stool examination.

    c. Checking of vital signs, most especially BP.

    d. Liver function test.

10. Nurse Pia is caring for a cancer patient that receives subcutaneous morphine to alleviate pain. Nurse Pia knows that it is important to monitor:

    a. Urine output

    b. Respiratory rate

    c. Heart rate

    d. Blood pressure

11. The school nurse endorsed a patient to the emergency room department after a fall in the basketball game. The school nurse said that she just stabilize the foot with a splint. After the routine triage, what is the next intervention to be done?

    a. Prepare hot water bag and place on the injured leg.

    b. Secure the leg using an elastic bandage.

    c. Anticipate an order for X-ray.

    d. Anticipate and prepare pain medication.

12. The physician prescribed $MgSO_4$ to a pregnant patient due to pre-eclampsia. The nurse knows that the IM route for the medication is:

    a. Deltoid muscles

    b. Vastus lateralis site

    c. Ventrogluteal site

    d. Dorsogluteal site

13. In question #12, the dorsogluteal site can be found by dividing the right gluteal muscle into four quadrants and is located in:

    a. Upper left quadrant

    b. Upper right quadrant

    c. Lower left quadrant

    d. Lower right quadrant

14. The nurse immediately calls the attention of the physician because of the patient has developed pulmonary embolism. Which of the following observation leads to the notion?

    a. The patient exhibits hypersomnolence and decrease interaction to the relatives.

    b. All of a sudden the patient complains of chest pain and shortness of breath.

    c. The patient suddenly complains of pain in his abdomen and is grimacing.

    d. The patient suddenly has chills and difficulty of eating.

15. The nurse is doing a skin test of cephalexin on a patient. Which of the following is the best part to perform the test:

    a. On the abdomen, two inches away from the umbilicus.

    b. On the lateral part of the femoral area.

    c. On the dorsal part of the arm near the elbow.

    d. On the hairless part of the forearm.

16. A patient suspected of Hodgkin's lymphoma is admitted to the oncology unit. Which of the following symptoms is likely associated with this disease?

    a. Painful cervical lymph nodes

    b. Night sweats and fatigue

    c. Nausea and vomiting

    d. Rapid respiration and weight gain

17. A mother in the well-baby clinic asks the nurse, "What will I do if my baby still asks for a bottle of milk at night?" The nurse's best response is:

    a. "It is okay to give the child another of a bottle of milk."

    b. "Perhaps it would be better if you change is with a glass of juice instead."

    c. "It is best to give him a bottle of water instead of milk."

    d. "Whatever happens, do not give another bottle of milk."

18. The patient admitted due to abdominal problems is ready for discharge. Nurse Vic is in charge of giving the health teachings to the client. The following is the correct health teachings regarding decreasing the occurrence of constipation, EXCEPT:

   a. Increase fiber in the diet.

   b. Advise the client to take laxative as needed.

   c. Drink at least 6-8 glasses of water every day.

   d. Having at least 30 minutes of exercise every day.

19. The nurse is mixing NPH and Regular insulin. Here are the following steps:
   I. After withdrawing the ordered amount of regular insulin, remove the syringe and expel any air bubbles.
   II. Pressurize NPH vial with an amount of air equal to the amount of NPH to be mixed with regular insulin and then remove the syringe.
   III. Inject remaining air into regular insulin vial and then withdraw the amount of regular insulin into the syringe.
   IV. Reinsert syringe into NPH vial and withdraw ordered amount of NPH.
   What is the sequence?

   a. i, ii, iii, iv

   b. ii, iii, i, iv

   c. iii, i, ii, iv

   d. i, iii, ii, iv

20. In the emergency department, the nurse is challenged on her prioritization skills. That is the reason beyond triage, to be able to detect the patient needing the most care. Among the following patient, who should receive the highest priority?

   a. A patient with headache, abdominal cramps, and intermittent fever for the past 48 hours.

   b. A patient with bruising on the right foot, unable to step, due to a sports competition.

   c. A patient with complaints of chest pain and abdominal pain after having dinner.

d. A patient with an approximately one inch laceration on the forehead due to accidental bump.

21. A patient suspected of bowel obstruction has a nasogastric tube attached to low suction. The nurse anticipates an arterial blood gas result of:

a. pH 7.50, pCO_2 55 mmHg

b. pH 7.40, pCO_2 40 mmHg

c. pH 7.20, pCO_2 25 mmHg

d. pH 7.35, pCO_2 35 mmHg

22. A patient is admitted to the surgical unit for cholecystectomy. A history reveals that the patient is taking in Coumadin oral as part of her medicine for her heart problem. As the nurse in charge of the patient, what should you anticipate as the next action in this process?

a. An order to withdraw blood samples for prothrombin (PT) and international normalize ratio (INR) level.

b. An order to administer vitamin K to the patient.

c. Prepare for transfusion, by drawing a sample for crossmatching.

d. Prepare patient for discharge as the surgery will not be done.

23. The patient was ordered by the patient to undergo some lab testing to be presented on her next follow-up check-up. During the follow-up of the patient, while waiting for his turn in the consulting unit, he asks the nurse, "What do you think about my lab results?" Looking at the result, which of the following are abnormal? (NOTE: there is more than one answer)

a. Hemoglobin 10 g/dL

b. Total cholesterol 300 mg/dL

c. Total serum protein 7 g/dL

d. Glycosylated hemoglobin A1C 5.4%

24. The nurse is giving Humulin R insulin to a diabetic patient. The nurse knows that Humulin R is the only kind of insulin that:

    a. Can be given subcutaneously.

    b. Can be given intravenously.

    c. Can be mixed with other insulins

    d. Can be mixed with antibiotics.

25. The nurse is giving health teachings to mothers regarding cerebral palsy. Which of the following information should be included in her teaching? (NOTE: there is more than one answer)

    a. Importance of regular developmental screening.

    b. The development of cerebral palsy and the causes.

    c. Delay on developmental stages with no needed intervention is normal.

    d. Importance of support groups for sharing.

26. A patient is admitted to the surgical unit for a diagnostic exam. One of the exams is a liver biopsy. The following exams test coagulation of the blood, EXCEPT:

    a. Hemoglobin count

    b. Partial prothrombin time

    c. Prothrombin time

    d. Platelet count

27. A patient in the cardiac unit on telemetry monitoring suddenly goes into ventricular fibrillation. The code team was alerted and prepares to defibrillate. Which of the following states the correct placement of the conducive gel pads?

    a. Right clavicle and left lower sternum.

    b. Left clavicle and right lower sternum.

    c. Right side of the sternum, below the clavicle and left of the precordium.

    d. Left side of the sternum, below the clavicle and right of the precordium.

28. Nurse A is supervising a new nurse B in assessing the abdomen of a patient. Upon auscultation, nurse B reports that she hears "gurgles" in all quadrants, but hears "swishing" sounds in only two quadrants. Nurse A explains that:

    a. The patient has an abnormality in the two quadrants that needs further assessment.

    b. The case of the patient affects the bowel sounds heard by nurse B.

    c. The frequency and intensity of the bowel sounds vary depending on the phase of digestion.

    d. Nurse B needs to reassess the bowel sounds of the patient.

29. A patient arrives in the emergency room department due to pain in his eyes. He reported that he accidentally splashed his eye with a household cleaner while doing home chores. The ER nurse should:

    a. Cover the eye with a sterile gauze or a patch.

    b. Irrigate the eye continuously with a sterile normal saline solution.

    c. Administer fluorescein drops in the affected eye.

    d. Assess by using a penlight and check visual acuity.

30. A nurse received a patient from the operating room that underwent hip replacement surgery. Which of the following assessment should alert the nurse?

    a. Complaints of pain upon positioning.

    b. Scanty blood discharge in the dressing.

    c. Careful movement of the patient.

    d. Temperature of 102°F (38.8°C).

31. A mother rushed her son in the hospital due to uncontrolled seizure disorder. The nurse anticipates the physician's orders which includes the following, EXCEPT:

    a. Administer Phenytoin IV 1.25mg/kg every 5 minutes.

    b. Restrain the patient's limbs during seizure.

    c. Position the patient on his side with head flexed.

    d. Notify the physician immediately.

32. The patient is complaining about his IV insertion site, he wants it to be removed by the nurse. Upon assessment, the nurse suspects infiltration. Which of the following supports this notion?

   a. Red line along course of the vein.

   b. Swelling, redness and tenderness of the site.

   c. Swelling, blanching of the skin and cool to touch.

   d. Redness and rashes around the tape.

33. The nurse is giving health teachings to a patient with renal disease regarding the typical side effects of corticosteroids. Which of the following should not be included?

   a. Cushingoid features.

   b. Hypertension

   c. Weight gain

   d. Hyponatremia

34. The nurse notes phlebitis in the IV insertion site of one patient. Which of the following should the nurse do first?

   a. Apply warm compress to the site.

   b. Discontinue IV.

   c. Insert IV in a new site.

   d. Flush the IV line with normal saline.

35. A nurse in a community outreach is discussing to mothers about the importance of immunizations for their children. Which of the following statements provides the most accurate information?

   a. All known infectious diseases can be prevented by specifically formulated immunizations.

   b. Immunizations are used to provide natural immunity against diseases for the young.

   c. In an attempt to minimize all diseases, immunizations are made to be risk-free and given universally.

d. Immunizations are used to provide acquired immunity from some specific diseases.

36. A patient was rushed to the hospital after a bee sting. The nurse observes that the patient has rashes in the body, redness and oral swelling. What is the most important nursing diagnosis for the patient?

    a. Risk for ineffective respiratory function

    b. Risk for ineffective tissue perfusion

    c. Disturbed body image

    d. Impaired oral mucous membrane

37. The clinic nurse receives a call from a mother whose son has ADHD. She told the nurse, "I am worried that my son is experiencing some side effects from the medicine." The nurse should address the problem by telling the nurse that the one of the side effects is:

    a. Increase in weight.

    b. Sleepiness.

    c. Agitation.

    d. Increase in appetite.

38. A patient with schizophrenia on home care and therapy is taking Haloperidol. She phoned the clinic to report that she is experiencing some movements in her face and tongue, which she believes is abnormal. The nurse knows that this is a symptom of:

    a. Hallucinations

    b. Co-morbid depression

    c. Pseudo-parkinsonism

    d. Tardive dyskinesia

39. The nurse is teaching a newly diagnosed diabetes mellitus patient regarding signs of hypoglycemia. Which of the following responses of the patient indicates understanding?

    a. "It includes confusion and lightheadedness."

    b. "It includes polydipsia and shakiness."

c. "It includes blurred vision and nervousness."

d. "It includes polyphagia, and dizziness."

40. A patient with COPD (Chronic Obstructive Pulmonary Disease) was rushed to the hospital after 3 days of worsening symptoms. A measurement of arterial blood gas revealed pH-7.3, $PaCO_2$-67 mmHg, HCO_3-29 mmol/L, PaO_2- 62 mmHg. The nurse interprets this as:

a. Respiratory Alkalosis, Partially compensated

b. Respiratory Acidosis, Partially compensated

c. Metabolic Alkalosis, Fully compensated

d. Metabolic Acidosis, Partially compensated

41. A 7-year old patient diagnosed with Wilm's tumor stage II, was admitted for treatment. The nurse knows that this stage is:

a. Cancer is limited to the kidneys and can be completely removed by surgery.

b. Cancer has spread to the areas surrounding the kidney and can be completely removed by surgery.

c. Cancer has spread to the areas surrounding the kidneys or other nearby organs and can be completely removed by surgery.

d. Cancer has spread beyond the area of the kidney into other organs.

42. A patient with difficulty of urinating and pain in the lower back was admitted to the renal unit. The doctor suspects acute glomerulonephritis. The following signs are related to the disease, EXCEPT:

a. Generalized edema

b. Urine specific gravity-1.040

c. Urine output for 24 hours-300ml

d. Brown urine

43. With question #42, which of the following can be a cause of acute glomerulonephritis?

a. Post-streptococcal infection.

b. Congenital condition and renal problem as complication.

c. Nephrotic syndrome.

d. Increase acidity of the blood.

44. The nurse checks the records of one patient with respiratory alkalosis. The nurse knows that this information shows the correct diagnosis, as the common causes of respiratory alkalosis includes: (Note: there are more than one answer)

a. Hyperventilation

b. Renal failure

c. Anxiety

d. Diabetic Ketoacidosis

45. The patient is telling the nurse that she never had any sexual contact nor has been injected, and can't accept how she was diagnosed with Hepatitis A. The nurse knows that Hepatitis A is most likely because:

a. The nature of her job.

b. Contaminated food.

c. Use of illegal drug.

d. Having pricked by a needle when sewing.

46. A leukemia patient is in need of blood after chemotherapy. A relative offered to share his blood and history was taken and he is assessed. Which of the following will assessment will likely prevent him from being a donor?

a. He was a dengue patient, 4 years ago.

b. He has Hepatitis C, 7 years ago.

c. He had cholecystectomy a year ago.

d. He is having an exercise therapy.

47. The nurse is having a ward class in the surgery ward about cholecystitis. The nurse teaches them regarding the necessary diet. Which of the following is the correct statement?

   a. It should be a low caloric diet.

   b. A high protein, low carbohydrate diet.

   c. The diet should be less glucose, less salt.

   d. It should be decreased in fatty foods.

48. A nurse is doing her routine vital signs checking on a patient taking Propranolol (Inderal). Which of the following indicates a side effect of the drug?

   a. Dry oral mucosa

   b. Bradycardia

   c. Paresthesia

   d. Urinary retention

49. A patient in the coronary unit is admitted due to Jervell and Lange-Nielsen syndrome. As part of monitoring and treatment, the physician orders ECG. The result shows:

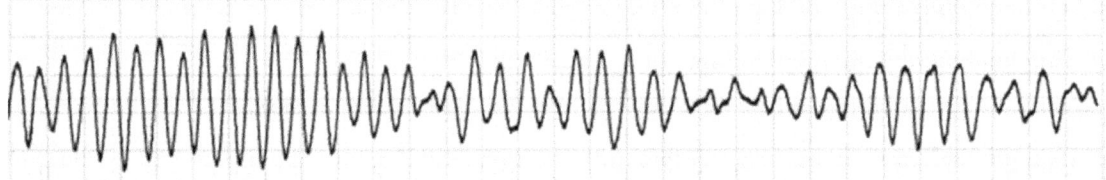

   a. Ventricular Tachycardia Monomorphic

   b. Ventricular Tachycardia Polymorphic

   c. Torsade de Pointes

   d. Asystole

50. A nurse is evaluating a 24 hours post-operative patient in wound healing. During assessment, the nurse noted that there is the presence of moderate amounts of serous drainage on the dressing. What is the next action of the nurse?

   a. Notify the physician.

b. Administer topical antibiotic on the wound.

c. Remove the dressing and air dry the wound.

d. Change the dressing and document.

51. The nurse receives a patient status post fiberglass cast application for a fractured right arm. She then gives teaching to the patient regarding the signs needed to be reported immediately. Which of the following shows his understanding?

    a. "I should report any itchiness under my cast."

    b. "I should report pain in my right shoulder."

    c. "I should report pain in my lower right arm."

    d. "I should report a warm sensation in my fingers."

52. One function of a nurse to monitor the dietary intake of their patient. During a home visit to an elderly male with a sedentary lifestyle, how many calories should he have?

    a. 2800

    b. 1600

    c. 2400

    d. 2000

53. An elderly patient with osteoarthritis is ready for discharge. The nurse is preparing her discharge teachings. Which of the following should be included?

    a. Include in the activities of daily living the physical activities and moderate exercises to decrease the discomfort felt by the patient.

    b. Resting the affected leg every night will heal the joint.

    c. The patient can drink non-steroidal analgesic without regards to food.

    d. The patient should already plan to enter a physical therapy session after discharge.

54. An elderly patient was brought to the nursing home. Upon assessment, the patient is observed to have the following symptoms: very thin, with muscle wasting and shows weakening health condition. The nurse suspects, which of the following:

    a. Venous stasis

    b. Catabolism

    c. Cachexia

    d. Malnutrition

55. The physician is adding new orders for a patient with osteoporosis, which is a medication of Alendronate (Fosamax). The nurse should question the order if:

    a. The patient has hypertension and on ACE inhibitor therapy.

    b. The patient has an allergy to shellfish or seafood.

    c. The patient is on low calorie/low carbohydrate diet.

    d. The patient is on complete bed rest and must remain supine.

56. The patient will undergo cataract surgery and the nurse is preparing the patient. The patient told the nurse how nervous he is. The nurse knows that in order to decrease anxiety and post surgical discomfort, it is important to:

    a. Give preoperative teaching.

    b. Give the preoperative checklist.

    c. Give psychological counselling.

    d. Give the necessary preoperative medication.

57. The nurse in a community assembly is discussing the ways to prevent Lyme disease. The following statements are ways of prevention, EXCEPT:

    a. Application of insect repellent on skin and clothes.

    b. Wearing long sleeve clothe and long pants.

    c. Drinking prophylactic antibiotic therapy.

    d. Careful assessment of the skin and hair for ticks.

58. A 1-year old pediatric patient suddenly went into cardiac arrest. In order to properly assess the pulse of the patient, the nurse knows that it is to check the:

    a. Radial pulse

    b. Brachial pulse

    c. Pedal pulse

    d. Carotid pulse

59. A patient received blood transfusion of 2 units PRBC for treatment of anemia. After a few hours, the nurse checks on the patient and saw her sitting on the bed, has a difficulty of breathing, and seems irritable. The nurse auscultated for lung sounds and heard crackles in the lower lobes of both lungs. Which of the following indicates such symptoms?

    a. Hemolytic reaction

    b. Febrile non-hemolytic reaction

    c. Allergic reaction

    d. Fluid overload

60. The nurse is teaching a patient on the proper way of deep breathing exercise and coughing exercises while sitting down. The nurse knows that the patient should sit upright because:

    a. It is physically comfortable.

    b. It helps the patient breath better.

    c. It helps loosen respiratory secretions.

    d. It helps the nurse observe the patient.

61. A nurse is caring for a pregnant patient in the labor unit that received amniotomy. Which of the following indicates understanding of the procedure? (Note: there is more than one answer)

    a. The nurse needs to frequently monitor the patient's cervical dilation after the procedure.

    b. The patient's contraction may become stronger after the procedure.

c. The nurse needs to monitor fetal heart rate closely after the procedure.

d. The patient will not feel discomfort during the procedure.

62. Looking at the ECG strip below, the nurse understands that this is:

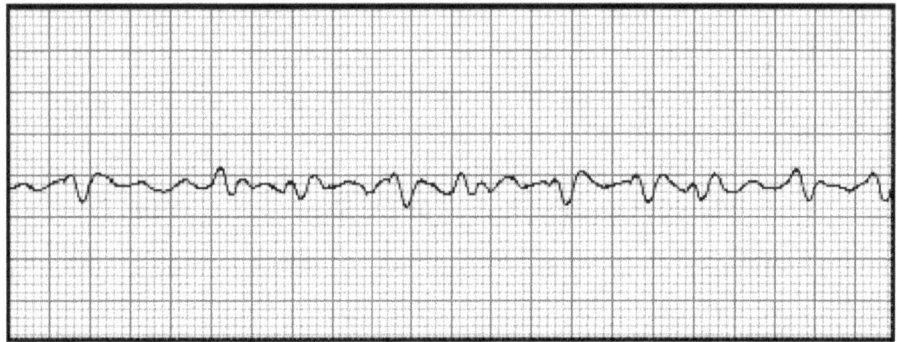

   a. Atrial Tachycardia

   b. Ventricular Tachycardia

   c. Atrial Fibrillation

   d. Ventricular Fibrillation

63. A grade school student was rushed to the hospital after school due to vomiting and unresponsiveness. Assessment reveals Kussmaul breathing, lethargy, irritability as response to stimuli, sunken eyes and dry mucous membranes. History reveals polydipsia, polyuria and bed wetting in the last two weeks. ABG was done and revealed: pH-7.10, PaO_2-92 mmHg, $PaCO_2$-30 mmHg, and HCO_3-16 mmol/L. This shows:

   a. Respiratory Acidosis, Uncompensated

   b. Metabolic Acidosis, Uncompensated

   c. Respiratory Acidosis, Partially Compensated

   d. Metabolic Acidosis, Partially Compensated

64. The nurse is preparing discharge instructions to a post-partum mother with an infant with hyperbilirubinemia. Which of the following should NOT be included in the information given?

   a. The mother should frequently do breastfeeding, preferably every 2 to 4 hours.

   b. The mother should adhere to the follow-up check-up after 72 hours.

c. Teach the mother regarding the signs of dehydration.

d. Make sure that the baby is placed in a quiet room, in a bassinet with dim light.

65. During the afternoon shift on the 2 east unit, a fire drill is being conducted. As the nurse, you are instructed to follow a horizontal evacuation plan. Where will you evacuate your patients?

a. On the lower floor, 2 east.

b. On the same floor, 2 west.

c. On the lower floor, 2 west.

d. On the same floor, 3 east.

66. The patient diagnosed with myocardial infarction and is recovering was instructed by his physician to ambulate in the hallways as part of his leg exercises. The nurse knows that this is because:

a. To eliminate the boredom of the patient.

b. To prevent pressure ulcers.

c. To help him get back in shape and increase physical activity.

d. To prevent deep vein thrombosis.

67. A patient has hypomagnesemia and requires supplemental magnesium. The nurse knows that magnesium:

a. Is the most abundant negatively charged ion in the extracellular fluid.

b. Is the most abundant positively charged ion in the extracellular fluid.

c. Assists in the acid-base regulation.

d. Is essential for enzyme and neurochemical activities.

68. A patient was rushed to the hospital with symptoms of myocardial infarction. Upon observation, the nurse suspects progression of the patient to cardiogenic shock. Which of the following supports this notion?

a. Extremely high blood pressure, 40 mmHg from the patient's normal systolic.

b. Pulse rate <60 bpm.

c. Bounding and rapid pulse.

d. Confusion.

69. A nurse overhears an LPN talking to a patient in an abusive manner. Checking it, the nurse saw that the LPN is holding the hand of the patient while talking to him in a non-therapeutic manner. The nurse should:

a. Call the security officer to arrest the LPN.

b. Report the act to the charge nurse.

c. Investigate further by asking the patient.

d. Do nothing because, it was just a misunderstanding.

70. A patient who became unconscious was brought by a stranger to the emergency department. The health care team performed the necessary interventions for the patient. The health care team can perform such interventions because of what consent?

a. Involuntary

b. Expressed

c. Implied

d. Informed

71. Patient X fell unconscious and hit her head on the ground while enjoying a party and drinking some beer. Her friend Carl dialled "911." Upon the arrival of the rescue team, assessment findings reveal that patient X has shallow and slow respirations, tachycardia, with profuse bleeding from both ears. The patient is at risk of what acid-base balance?

a. Respiratory Acidosis

b. Respiratory Alkalosis

c. Metabolic Acidosis

d. Metabolic Alkalosis

72. The nurse is discussing the modifiable and hereditary risk factors of atherosclerosis. The patient understands the hereditary risk factors by responding:

    a. "The risk increases due to family history of heart diseases."

    b. "I need to decrease my weight."

    c. "I have to quit smoking."

    d. "The risk increases as I age."

73. The nurse believes that a patient in any case needs to adapt to the changes in their lifestyle and to their environment to help them prevent and/or treat their diseases. This Adaptation Theory of nursing practice is the concept of:

    a. Madeleine Leininger

    b. Dorothea Orem

    c. Sister Callista Roy

    d. Martha Rogers

74. A teenager refuses to join their physical education class and tells his teacher that he has a condition. The teacher asks the child to bring a letter from his doctor to prove this. The next day, the student gave a medical certificate to his teacher due to Osgood-Schlatter disease. The teacher went to the school clinic to ask the nurse about the disease. The nurse answers:

    a. "It is just a form escape from the physical activities of the school, nothing to worry about."

    b. "The student is scheduled for a surgery on his left knee."

    c. "The student experiences discomfort and swelling of the inferior aspect of the knee."

    d. "The student has a weak bone that may fracture easily during physical activities."

75. The nurse talks to the patient and ask for some information, she also talks to the family members who is with the family to gather and validate the information. This process is done in which of phase of the nursing process?

    a. The evaluation phase

b. The implementation phase

c. The planning phase

d. The assessment phase

76. A mother went to the Under-five Clinic. His 4-year old son is having high fever and rashes in the body. The nurse assessing the patient saw lesions that look like "teardrops on a rose petal." This characteristic is found in:

a. Measles

b. Allergy

c. Chicken pox

d. Eczema

77. The nurse is evaluating the patient with pneumonia for the effectiveness of the nursing care plan. Which of the following statements shows that the objective was reached?

a. "At the end of the shift, the nurse will be able to provide adequate hydration for the patient."

b. "At the end of the shift, the nurse will be able to ensure patient safety as manifested by no falls and injuries."

c. "At the end of the shift, the patient will be able to perform deep breathing and coughing exercises every 2 hours."

d. "At the end of the shift, the patient will be able to value the care and interventions provided for his health."

78. The physician has an order of Heparin 6,880 units to be given Sub Q OD. The available stock is 10,000 units per ml. How much should the nurse give?

a. 0.68 ml

b. 1.68 ml

c. 0.16 ml

d. 1.16 ml

79. The nurse attends a seminar regarding malpractices done by healthcare professionals and the equivalent punishment for the offenses. The nurse understands that an action is called malpractice when it has the following elements:

I. A breach of duty

II. An intentional act

III. Foreseeability

IV. Patient harm

V. Causation

  a. i, ii, iii, iv

  b. i, ii, iii, v

  c. i, iii, iv, v

  d. ii, iii, iv, v

80. A mother brought her child for a follow-up check-up due to his asthma. One of the medications prescribed previously was Diphenhydramine (Benadryl) to be taken in 3 times a day. The nurse asks how much is the dose, and she said the doctor explained that it should be 5mg/kg/day and gave the child 25mg every intake. The nurse knows what the dose for a child weighing 30kg should be, and concluded that the intake of the child is:

  a. The correct dose.

  b. Too low.

  c. Too high.

  d. Not flexible, it should depend on the symptoms.

81. The nurse in the operating room is preparing a sterile field. The nurse knows that she should stop preparing only if:

  a. When the nurse placed the sterile item 1 inch instead of 2 inches from the edge of the sterile field.

  b. When the nurse finished setting the field, this should be done in a continuous process.

  c. When the nurse prepared the sterile solution in the sterile container.

d. When the nurse turns her upper body away from the field because the surgeon calls her.

82. You are the charge nurse in the orthopedic ward giving assignments for the day. A nurse from the medical ward was floated to your unit. Which of the following patients should be assigned to her?

    a. A patient with a fiberglass cast with numbness and discoloration of toes.

    b. A patient on skeletal traction who needs assistance in ADLs.

    c. A patient 1 day post-operative of above the knee amputation, with fever of 100.8°F in the previous shift.

    d. A patient 48 hours post-operative of total hip replacement, on glucose monitoring.

83. An occupational health nurse is attending to a patient with Avulsed tooth. What should the nurse do to preserve the tooth, in case it can be implanted?

    a. Place it in a normal saline.

    b. Place it in cold water.

    c. Place it in milk.

    d. Place it in clean, warm water.

84. A patient went to the emergency room department after a radiologic incident. What intervention should be prioritized?

    a. Decontamination of the patient's clothes.

    b. Decontamination of the patient's open wound.

    c. Decontamination of the examination room used by the patient.

    d. Decontamination of the equipment used for the patient.

85. A nurse is taking care of a Japanese patient. During the assessment, the nurse greeted the patient. Which of the following should the nurse perform to build rapport?

    a. The nurse should maintain direct eye contact with the patient.

    b. The nurse should stay near the patient.

c. The nurse should touch the patient's hand as often as possible.

d. The nurse should greet the patient in a formal manner.

86. The nurse is caring for a 4-year old pediatric patient diagnosed with cystic fibrosis. The nurse knows that to care for the patient, she must also understand the developmental task of the patient, which is:

a. To be able to learn the deep breathing and coughing exercises in a fun manner.

b. To establish his own industry and self-confidence.

c. To develop his autonomy and self-control in making choices for his plan of care.

d. To develop his initiative and sense of purpose.

87. The nurse receives a patient from the post anesthesia care unit. The nurse should give first priority to:

a. The patient's respiratory status.

b. The patient's level of consciousness.

c. The patient's discomfort and level of pain.

d. The patient's reflexes and ability to move peripheries.

88. According to Maslow's Hierarchy of needs, every individual has 5 levels of needs, starting from Physiological Needs. Which of the following shows the correct order of the other levels?

I. Self-esteem

II. Self-actualization

III. Psychological needs

IV. Love and belongingness

a. iii, iv, i, ii

b. iii, i, ii, iv

c. iv, iii, ii, i

d. iv, ii, i, iii

89. The nurse is preparing a patient for Colposcopy. The doctor explained that the patient needs to undergo to examine her insides better. Which of the following should the nurse do first?

    a. Reiterate to the patient the information that the doctor explained, to alleviate her anxiety.

    b. Assist the patient with the application of the silver nitrate medication to control the bleeding.

    c. Discuss with the patient the importance of regular douche.

    d. Administer pain medications as prescribed by the physician.

90. A primigravida mother is excited for her first monthly check-up and asks the nurse, "When does my baby's heart pump its own blood?" The nurse response is based on the knowledge that this happens during:

    a. 5th week

    b. 3rd week

    c. 6th week

    d. 9th week

91. The wife of a Puerto Rican geriatric patient approaches the nurse and told her that she cannot sign the consent for surgery. The nurse understands that their customs dictate that:

    a. She needs to consult her husband first.

    b. She does not know how to write.

    c. She cannot sign by law.

    d. She needs to ask the children and relatives first.

92. The nurse is in charge of 4 patients in the medical-surgical unit. During her regular rounds, who among them should be seen first?

    a. The patient with diabetes preparing for discharge today.

b. The patient with tracheotomy reported by the previous shift to have copious secretions.

c. The patient with a schedule for physical therapy this morning.

d. The patient with pressure ulcers in needs of dressing change.

93. A nurse is assigned to discuss the symptoms of cancer to a group of community people. One of the participants asked the nurse, "Which of the following cancer has the poorest prognosis?" The nurse responds:

a. Skin cancer

b. Gastric cancer

c. Breast cancer

d. Pancreatic cancer

94. At the end of the shift, nurse Paul is walking in the hallway when he accidentally peeps on one ward and saw a patient lying on the floor. What should he do?

a. Call the next shift nurse; it's not his responsibility anymore.

b. Determine whether the patient is responsive.

c. Help the patient back to bed.

d. Call for help.

95. A geriatric patient was admitted to the hospital due to persistent vomiting for 2 days. Assessment reveals lethargy and myalgia, dry mucous membrane, capillary refill of greater than 4 seconds. Arterial Blood Gas results are: pH-7.7, PaO_2-75 mmHg, $PaCO_2$-45 mmHg, HCO_3-34 mmol/L. This is known as an acid-base imbalance of:

a. Respiratory Alkalosis, Uncompensated

b. Respiratory Alkalosis, Fully Compensated

c. Metabolic Alkalosis, Uncompensated

d. Metabolic Alkalosis, Partially Compensated

96. A pregnant patient insists that she can deliver her baby via normal spontaneous delivery. However, the physician explained that it is necessary for her size, and her hips are small to deliver normally. The nurse knows that cesarean section is mostly the choice for this kind of hips:

    a. Anthropoid hips
    b. Android hips
    c. Platypelloid hips
    d. Gynecoid hips

97. During the night shift, a nursing assistant working with Nurse Pat tells him that one of the nurses in the unit is not assessing the patient, regardless of the request of the patient. Nurse Pat should:

    a. Confront the nurse to know if the nursing assistant is telling the truth.
    b. Talk to the patient who is requesting to investigate.
    c. Tell the nursing assistant shouldn't do that.
    d. Contact the nursing supervisor about the situation.

98. After a diagnostic procedure, the physician tells the patient that she has a "Mallory-Weiss" tear. During the rounds, the patient tells the nurse that she did not understand what "Mallory-Weiss" tear is. The nurse tells the patient that it is:

    a. A kind of diverticulosis, found in the intestines.
    b. An esophageal tear that can be caused by alcohol drinking.
    c. A lacrimal gland disorder, so the patient will not be able to produce tears.
    d. A tear caused by peptic ulcer.

99. A nurse in a home-care facility is reviewing the history of one elderly patient. She notes the different immunizations given to her. Which of the following should be the priority?

    a. Hepa A vaccine
    b. Mumps vaccine
    c. Hepa B vaccine

d. Pneumoccocal vaccine

100. A nurse is giving lectures to new nursing assistants regarding infection control, most especially hand washing techniques. Which of the following demonstrate a correct teaching?

   a. Hand washing should be done within one minute using soap and running water.

   b. Hand washing should be done within two minutes using soap and running water.

   c. Hand washing should be done using hot water so that the natural fats in the skin will be emulsified.

   d. Hand washing should be done using cold water so that the natural fats in the skin will be emulsified.

ANSWERS:

1. Correct Answer: C.

To prevent medication errors, the nurse should always have a second nurse witness when mixing insulin and double-check dose and type of insulin that needs to be administered.

2. Correct Answer: C.

The primary nursing intervention the nurse should perform upon the arrival of a patient in the emergency room department is to take the vital signs. This will serve as a baseline of further diagnosing tests. Medical history can be done after taking the vital signs to understand more about the condition of the patient.

3. Correct Answer: C.

Being culturally-sensitive environment is important to the most possible way in accordance with the hospital policy, without disrupting nursing routines. Traditional rituals and food is needed in their beliefs in order to help them welcome the situation with whole heartedly. Restricting them in doing their traditions will not complete the transition from life to death.

4. Correct Answer: A.

The charge nurse should give an assignment based on the knowledge and experience of the nurse to handle the situation. For the floated nurse, coming from the labor unit will have limited knowledge in taking care of patients in the cardiac unit. Therefore the most stable patient should be considered. This is exhibited by the patient in choice A, the patient is stable and is ready for discharge.

5. Correct Answer: B.

Glucagon is a hormone that works in opposite from insulin, both are hormones produced by the pancreas. Therefore, if the patient's sugar level drops unwantedly, glucagon should be given to reverse the process.

6. Correct Answer: D.

A patient with symptoms of vomiting and diarrhea is at risk of fluid and electrolyte imbalance. The best IV solution to this situation is a multielectrolyte solution such as LR. This will treat dehydration and restore normal fluid balance.

7. Correct Answer: A.

The most prominent sign that a mother can observe if the diuretic given is no longer effective is the sudden weight gain of the baby. This is due to fluid accumulation.

8. Correct Answer: B.

The therapeutic blood level of Phenytoin is 10 -20 mcg/ml. Therefore, among the choices, B is the lowest, while choices A, C, and D are in normal range.

9. Correct Answer: D.

Hepatic toxicity and damage is the result of acetaminophen toxicity, and if not diagnosed and treated can lead to death. The nurse should anticipate N-acetylcysteine administration as the antidote.

10. Correct Answer: B.

Morphine sulfate is an opioid analgesic with a narcotic effect as a side effect, it can cause respiration and respiratory reflex suppression. Therefore, the nurse should monitor the patient's respiratory rate.

11. Correct Answer: C.

An X-ray should be ordered to rule-out fracture. This will guide the health workers on the next steps of treatment. Also, following the R-I-C-E therapy, cold compress is used, not hot compress. Compression such as an elastic bandage could be used if there is no fracture. Pain medication will depend on the need for the patient.

12. Correct Answer: D.

Deep intramuscular injections are given in the gluteal muscle, most particularly the dorsogluteal muscle. Choice A is the muscle below the acromial process, and is found in the upper part of the arm. Choice B is the muscle in the femur, the site for vit. K injection for pediatric patients. Choice C and D are both gluteal muscles, however, dorsogluteal site is the choice for $MgSO_4$ injections as it requires alternating buttocks.

13. Correct Answer: B.

The dorsogluteal muscle is also known as the "upper outer" quadrant. In the question, it shows the right gluteal muscle, therefore, its upper outer is the upper right quadrant.

14. Correct Answer: B.

The signs of pulmonary embolism are chest pain, shortness of breath and severe anxiety. If these are present the physician should be notified immediately. Pulmonary embolism has nothing to do with sleepiness (choice A), pain in the abdomen (choice C) and chills (choice D).

15. Correct Answer: D.

Skin test is done to test any allergic reaction to the medication using intradermal technique/angle. Intradermal injection site is on the forearm, clear from body hair, in order to check the reaction easily, if any. Choice A and B are for subcutaneous site. And choice C is not an injection site.

16. Correct Answer: B.

Hodgkin's lymphoma has the following symptoms: enlarged, but painless cervical lymph nodes, night sweats, fatigue, and tachycardia. Therefore, choices A, C, and D are not symptoms of Hodgkin's Lymphoma.

17. Correct Answer: C.

The risk for tooth decay increases because of drinking milk even when sleeping. To clean the sugar content in the child's mouth, it is best to give him a bottle of water. This will also result in decreasing the need of bottle at night, since the child will lose interest in the bottle.

18. Correct Answer: B.

The nurse should encourage the natural way of relieving constipation and not to rely on medications. Choices A, C and D are the best way to relieve constipation the natural way, and not choice B.

19. Correct Answer: B.

The nurse should consider the thickness of the insulin to be mixed together. In this case, NPH is thicker than Regular insulin. Therefore, Regular insulin should be withdrawn first following the correct way of aspirating medications in a vial.

20. Correct Answer: C.

The triage is designed to perform a quick assessment to prioritize the need of every patient and to know who needs further diagnosis and treatment. Following ABC, the patient in choice C falls the biggest need as it involves the heart. Included for those receiving first cares are airway problems, neurological and trauma.

21. Correct Answer: A.

A patient that has a nasogastric tube is at risk of metabolic alkalosis. This is the result of removing acids from the stomach. Among the choices, only choice A represents alkalosis. Choice B and C are acidosis, and choice D is within normal range.

22. Correct Answer: A.

In order to check if the patient is at risk of bleeding, the next order will be to get a sample for PT and INR. This will then dictate the next steps, if the patient needs vitamin K, or if the surgery will not take place. Choice C is only if there is bleeding.

23. Correct Answer: A and B.

The range for the normal hemoglobin is 12-16 g/dL. The total cholesterol should be <200 mg/dL to be considered normal. Choices C and D are within normal range.

24. Correct Answer: B.

Humulin R is a regular insulin. Regular insulins are the only kind that can be given intravenously (IV). Most insulins are given subcutaneously. There are other insulins that an be mixed together. However, insulins should not be mixed with antibiotics.

25. Correct Answer: A, B and D.

The nurse should be able to discuss the topics regarding the causes, sign and symptoms, treatment, and other interventions such as support groups to the mothers. Choice C should not be done; instead therapy is needed for the patient.

26. Correct Answer: A.

Choices B, C, and D are tests used to know the coagulation of the blood of the patient. Choice A deals with the red blood cells of the blood.

27. Correct Answer: C.

The conductive gel should follow the anatomy of the heart. Therefore, one pad should be placed on the right side of the sternum, just below the clavicle, the part of the heart where the signal starts. And the second pad placed on the left of the precordium.

28. Correct Answer: C.

Bowel sounds vary from one quadrant to another; some may have decreased vowel sound, while others increased. The sounds also vary, depending on the digestion and diseases in the abdomen.

29. Correct Answer: B.

The priority and emergency treatment of chemicals in the eye includes irrigation of the eye/s. It should be irrigated continuously for at least 10 minutes. Choice A will not relieve the pain and heal the eye. Choice C is to check the cornea for scratches. And choice D will be done after irrigating the eyes.

30. Correct Answer: D.

A patient post-surgery is at risk of infection due to break in the skin. Most especially for a patient post hip replacement, complications include neurovascular and infection. If the temperature given is a low-grade fever, then it is not a concern. Choices A and B are normal findings. While choice C is a normal reaction of the patient.

31. Correct Answer: B.

During the occurrence of the seizure disorder, the nurse should prioritize the safety of the patient and prevent aspiration. Safety can be promoted by putting up the side rails of the bed and ensuring the patient is lying down – not to restraint the limbs. Choice C will prevent aspiration. Choice A and D are also correct as it will help treat the patient.

32. Correct Answer: C.

Infiltration happens when the IV fluid can no longer pass through the catheter because it is blocked or kinked, as a result the fluids extravasates or leaks. This causes swelling, tenderness, decreased or no infusion rate, blanching of the skin and the site is cool to touch. Choice A and B are signs of Phlebitis. While choice D is irritation from the tape used.

33. Correct Answer: D.

Patients having corticosteroid therapy should be oriented on the typical side effects of the medicine in order for them not to panic. These are weight gain brought about by fluid retention, hypertension, Cushingoid features (the common one is moon face), Low serum albumin, and inflammatory response suppression. It also causes hypernatremia, not hyponatremia.

34. Correct Answer: B.

The first intervention for an IV site not working, such as in the case of phlebitis, is to discontinue and remove the IV line from the site. The next step is to place warm compress on the site, not a cold one. Then the nurse can now reinsert the IV line in a new site, preferable in the other hand/arm. The nurse should not attempt to flush the IV line as this will cause more pain and inflammation.

35. Correct Answer: D.

Immunization is made for some diseases, not all diseases have immunizations. This provides acquired immunity; natural immunity comes from the antibodies passed from the mother to the child. Like other medications, immunization cannot be considered as risk-free and there are things to consider before giving immunizations as presented by the WHO.

36. Correct Answer: A.

The patient might be experiencing an anaphylactic reaction that resulted in the signs and symptoms during the observation. The most important intervention should be to maintain the patency of the patient's airway as he can experience ineffective respiratory function. Other nursing diagnoses can follow as the treatment goes.

37. Correct Answer: C.

The side effects of the medication (CNS depressant) given for ADHD include: poor appetite, insomnia, and agitation.

38. Correct Answer: D.

Tardive dyskinesia is the involuntary and repetitive movements shown in the facial movements and tongue protrusion. Choices A, B, and C are also side effects of Haloperidol, but does not indicate the abnormal movements of the tongue and face.

39. Correct Answer: A.

The signs of hypoglycemia are shakiness, nervousness or anxiety, sweating, chills, clamminess, irritability, confusion, tachycardia, lightheadedness or dizziness, and hunger or nausea. Therefore, choices B, C, and D are incorrect.

40. Correct Answer: B.

The patient shows respiratory acidosis as seen by the increased carbon dioxide level. This can be a result of an acute exacerbation of COPD, and show partial compensation.

41. Correct Answer: B.

The staging depends on the area affected and is affected by surgery. Stage I is characterized by choice A. Stage II is characterized by choice B. Stage III is characterized by choice C. Stage IV is characterized by choice D.

42. Correct Answer: A.

Acute glomerulonephritis has the following symptoms: brown-colored urine (tea-colored or cola colored), foamy urine (protein in urine), hypertension, peri-orbital edema – not generalized, fatigue, the specific gravity is increased due to oliguria and blood in urine.

43. Correct Answer: A.

Glomerulonephritis can be caused by: post-streptococcal infection, examples are strep throat infection; bacterial endocarditis; and other immune diseases such as lupus.

44. Correct Answer: B.

The common causes of Respiratory Acidosis are asphyxia, respiratory and CNS depression, hyperventilation, anxiety and DKA. Renal failure is a cause of Metabolic Acidosis.

45. Correct Answer: B.

The nurse should explain to the patient that Hepatitis A is transmitted through contaminated food (fecal-oral route).

46. Correct Answer: B.

Hepatitis C is a kind of Hepatitis that is viral and is transmitted through bodily fluids that causes inflammation of the liver. A person with this kind of hepatitis can't donate blood due to the infection in his blood.

47. Correct Answer: D.

An inflammation of the gallbladder, responsible for the production of bile, which is necessary to digest fats in food. Therefore, the patient will have difficulty in digesting fats. The nurse should reiterate the importance of this diet.

48. Correct Answer: B.

Propranolol is a beta-blocker used to treat cardiac problems. However, precaution should be done when taking the medication. The nurse should always check for the pulse, as a <60 bpm indicates that the patient is experiencing side effects of the drug.

49. Correct Answer: C.

Torsade de Pointes is a kind of ventricular tachycardia characterized by difference in the amplitude of QRS and it looks like twisting around the baseline. The congenital causes include Jervell and Lange-Nielsen syndrome, and Romano-ward syndrome. Other causes include Acute Myocardial Infarction, Medications, Electrolyte imbalance, and Toxins.

50. Correct Answer: D.

The wound is healing properly, the moderate serous on the dressing shows that the wound is closing. The nurse should change the dressing and document that the wound's appearance is clean and healing. Choice A is not necessary. Choice B is not recommended, especially not ordered by the physician. And choice C needs to be done after 48-72 hours.

51. Correct Answer: C.

A pain in the lower arm of the affected part of the patient indicates impaired perfusion. This requires immediate removal of the cast to prevent further neurovascular compromise.

52. Correct Answer: D.

The 2000 calorie diet is recommended for older men with a sedentary lifestyle, active women and children. The nurse should also point out that in order to achieve this he should have 6 oz. of grains, 2 and a half cups of vegetables, 2 cups of fruits, and 3 cups of milk. Choice A is for active adults. Choice B is for sedentary women and children. And choice C is for sedentary adolescents.

53. Correct Answer: A.

The patient needs exercise and movement to help decrease the discomfort in the leg/joint. Most felt during waking up, in the morning, and decreases as the day pass as the patient moves.

54. Correct Answer: C.

Cachexia is a condition where the patient, mostly elderlies, suffer from ill health, malnutrition (seen in the body stature of the patient), and muscle wasting. Choice A refers to a blood disorder due to pooling of the blood in the vein. Choice B is the breakdown of tissue due to severe trauma or crush injuries. And choice D is the lack of nutrition in the patient.

55. Correct Answer: D.

Alendronate is a biphosphate used to treat and prevent osteoporosis for both men and women. It should not be given to patients that needs to complete bed rest and must remain supine because of its side effects. The patient needs to sit straight or upright for at least 30 minutes, and on an empty stomach, because it has gastrointestinal side effects, like esophageal irritation.

56. Correct Answer: A.

Preoperative patient teaching will help the patient understand the course of the surgery, what will happen and what to expect after. Choice B is a guide on how to prepare the patient before the procedure. Choice C is not necessary for a patient undergoing surgery. And choice D will not relieve anxiety and post surgical discomfort.

57. Correct Answer: C.

Prevention of Lyme disease is done by: wearing long pants and long sleeves; use of insect repellents; clearing of bush and lives in the yard; and check the skin and hair of family members and pets. It does not include taking of antibiotic as prophylaxis.

58. Correct Answer: B.

The brachial pulse is considered the most accessible and easy to palpate the site for infants. Choices A and C are not reliable for cardiac function due to being distant from the heart. Choice D will be difficult to palpate due to the fatty tissue surrounding the area.

59. Correct Answer: D.

Fluid overload happens when the body receives a fluid volume in a short period of time that the vascular system can't handle, this leads to leakage in the lungs. These are the symptoms: dyspnea, tachypnea, and irritable.

60. Correct Answer: B.

The patient should be in a sitting position when doing deep breathing and coughing exercises because it will help the lungs expand better, therefore helping the patient breath better. Choice A is incorrect as the most comfortable position is supine. Choice C is the effect of coughing exercises. Choice D is incorrect as interventions should be patient-centered not nurse-centered.

61. Correct Answer: B, C, and D.

Amniotomy is the artificial rupture of the membranes. The patient will not pain during the procedure and it is followed by a gush of amniotic fluid. After the procedure the nurse should monitor choices B and C. However, the cervical checks should be minimized to prevent infection.

62. Correct Answer: D.

Atrial and Ventricular difficulties can be separated by the QRS complex – in that Atrial has visible one, and Ventricular can't be recognized. Therefore the ECG strip shows a Ventricular problem. Ventricular Fibrillation is characterized as rapid and erratic heart's impulses. Ventricular Tachycardia is characterized as a fast or rapid heartbeat due to improper electrical activity of the heart with at least three irregular heartbeats in a row.

63. Correct Answer: D.

The patient has signs of Diabetes Mellitus as the history reveals and might be experiencing hypoglycemia. The pH indicates acidity, as well as his HCO_3 and PCO_2 levels. Following the rules of ABG, this indicates Metabolic Acidosis with partial compensation of the respiratory system.

64. Correct Answer: D.

A pediatric patient with Hyperbilirubinemia should be exposed to light (in a hospital setting, your blue/violet or UV light) to help process the bilirubin in the skin. The mother should know the importance of choices A, B and C for her child.

65. Correct Answer: B.

A horizontal evacuation plan means that the evacuation of the patients should be on the same floor of the corresponding opposite ward (east to west, vice versa; 1-1, 2-2 and so on). Choice A and C show a vertical evacuation plan.

66. Correct Answer: D.

A patient who has been in a supine position for a long time needs to ambulate to prevent deep vein thrombosis. The muscular contraction will help the veins to bring the blood back to the heart, and prevent hemostasis.

67. Correct Answer: D.

Magnesium is needed for enzyme and neurochemical activities and cardiac and muscular contraction. Choice A refers to Chlorine. Choice B refers to Potassium. Choice C refers to Phosphorus.

68. Correct Answer: D.

Cardiogenic shock happens when the heart becomes tired of pumping, therefore decrease in activity. As a result the blood cannot reach the vital organs and can manifest through symptoms affecting the brain, which is decreased LOC or confusion.

69. Correct Answer: B.

Nurses and other health practitioners are mandated by specific law (local and hospital policies) to report any incident to the charge nurse. Even if it is only suspected, it should be reported as the investigation will happen. The nurse will not be the rightful person responsible for the investigation. It is also incorrect to perform A and D as it involves care to the patient.

70. Correct Answer: C.

Implied consent refers to a presumption that an unconscious or mentally incapacitated patient would, under normal circumstances, consent to lifesaving treatment. Choice A is a consent to treat that is granted by law enforcement. Choice B is verbal, nonverbal gesturing or a written consent. And choice D is when the patient understands and agrees to the treatment.

71. Correct Answer: A.

The patient has shallow and slow breathing, which means that the respiratory is affected. It is acidosis due to the decrease exchange of oxygen to carbon dioxide. The shallow breathing will trap more CO_2.

72. Correct Answer: A.

Hereditary risk factors include those that can be passed from the parents to the child, such as heart diseases. Choice B, C, and D are modifiable risk factors that can be seen in a person's lifestyle.

73. Correct Answer: C.

Sister Callista Roy is the author of the Adaptation theory of nursing practice. Choice A developed Transcultural Nursing. Choice B developed the Self Care Model. And Choice D developed the Science of Unitary Human Beings theory.

74. Correct Answer: C.

Osgood-Schlatter disease happens due to continuous use of the quadriceps that presented with the symptoms: pain and swelling of the inferior aspect of the knee. Choice A is incorrect. Choice B is not necessary as this disease is self-limiting and can be treated. Choice C is seen osteogenesis imperfect.

75. Correct Answer: D.

Gathering of necessary information, such as the history, from the patient and the family members and validating the information should be done in the assessment phase. The information will then be used to perform the necessary intervention to heal the patient.

76. Correct Answer: C.

Chickenpox is characterized by a lesion that appears to be "teardrop on a rose petal." Choice A is characterized by small blue-white spots visible on the oral mucosa. Choice B may show redness and rashes, but no fever. Choice D is known for its patches appearance.

77. Correct Answer: C.

The outcome presented should be patient-centered, making choices A and B incorrect. The outcome should present a specific, measurable, achievable, realistic, and has a time frame, making choice D incorrect.

78. Correct Answer: A.

Following the formula Required over Stock multiplied by the Quantity will result to choice A.

79. Correct Answer: C.

The important elements of malpractice are: breach of duty, foreseeability, patient harm and causation. The breach of duty can be classified in an intentional act or non-intentional act.

80. Correct Answer: B.

To check the dosage the nurse should compute it: 5 x 30 = 150mg per day; 150 ÷ 3 = 50mg. Therefore, the patient should receive 50mg, 3 times a day, making the dose too low.

81. Correct Answer: D.

The nurse violated the sterile rule when she turns her upper body away from the field and must begin preparing a new sterile field. Choice A is the correct way of placing sterile things, the 1 inch rule. Choices B and C are also correct.

82. Correct Answer: D.

The most stable among the patients is choice D, also the need of monitoring the blood sugar is something the floater nurse is familiar of. Other choices need an experienced nurse in the orthopedic ward in order to monitor the patients very well.

83. Correct Answer: C.

An Avulsed tooth should be placed immediately in milk to preserve it to be ready for reimplantation. The nurse should also handle it from the crown and not the root.

84. Correct Answer: C.

The first priority should be to clean the patient's skin, especially the wound to limit the absorption of radiation in his body. Remember: patients first before the equipment.

85. Correct Answer: D.

The nurse should be aware of the Asian Heritage and Customs regarding communication. Japanese prefers to be greeted in a formal manner. Direct eye contact or invasion of personal space may cause uneasiness. And the nurse should touch the patient's hand only when necessary.

86. Correct Answer: D.

According to Erik Erikson's developmental Stages, a 4-year old child is in the initiative vs. guilt. He wants to develop a sense of purpose in what he does.

87. Correct Answer: A.

The nurse should give priority to the patient's respiratory status in accordance to the rule, "ABC."

88. Correct Answer: A.

According to Maslow's Hierarchy of Needs the proper order is: Physiological Needs, Safety and Psychological Needs, Love and Belongingness, Self-esteem, and Self-actualization.

89. Correct Answer: B.

The nurse need no longer explain what the doctor explained, making choice A incorrect. Choice C is not important at the time as it is information given as part of the discharge instructions. Choice D is incorrect as it is not part of preparing the patient. Choice B should be given priority because it will prevent and control the potential bleeding during the examination.

90. Correct Answer: B.

The embryonic heart starts pumping its own blood by the 3rd week, and the blood already has its own blood type. Choice A marks the development of the hands, legs, and the eyes, choice C marks the period where brain waves are already detectable. Choice D marks the development of teeth.

91. Correct Answer: A.

With regards to the health care practices of Puerto Rican people, the wife needs to consult the husband prior signing any consent. They may also require same-gender health care provider. It is not because of choices B, C, and D.

92. Correct Answer: B.

Checking for ABC is important in prioritization. Therefore, choice B must be assessed first to check the airway patency.

93. Correct Answer: D.

Among the types of cancer in the choices, pancreatic cancer is the only one asymptomatic until a surgical removal is needed for diagnosis. Therefore, it has the poorest diagnosis.

94. Correct Answer: B.

The nurse should first determine if the patient is conscious or unconscious. This will inform the next intervention that the nurse will do. Choice A is incorrect as it is still in the nurse's responsibility to promote care, even if it's no longer his shift. Choice C and D are incorrect as the nurse does not know what happened to the patient first.

95. Correct Answer: C.

The pH indicates alkalosis, $PaCO_2$ is normal, and HCO_3 is alkalosis. Therefore, it is Metabolic Alkalosis, uncompensated.

96. Correct Answer: B.

Android pelvis is characterized as heart-shaped hips that are common in 23% of women population. Choice A is oval shaped. Choice C is the flat hips, which is less common. And choice D is the round pelvis, which is the most common in women.

97. Correct Answer: D.

The nurse should address the problem following the proper channel of communication. Even if it's only a suspicion, the nurse should act. The nursing supervisor will be the person responsible in addressing the situation.

98. Correct Answer: B.

Mallory-Weiss syndrome is also known as Gastro-esophageal Laceration syndrome. It is a linear tear in the mucosa of the esophagus, particularly at the junction of esophagus and stomach.

99. Correct Answer: D.

An elderly is more prone to developing pneumonia, especially of the changes in the weather and those with chronic diseases. Therefore, the nurse should schedule the pneumococcal vaccine administration, which is usually given every 5 years.

100. Correct Answer: B.

The minimum minutes for hand washing is 2 minutes, some even teach to sing "Happy Birthday" and other songs for the "n^{th} time" just to make sure to reach the necessary time needed to wash the hands. It can be done using hot or cold water.